CREATION LIFE BIBLE EXPLORATION

A Journey of Discovery

CREATION Life

EDITOR IN CHIEF Robyn Edgerton

AUTHOR Chris Blake

RESEARCHER Heather Neal

CONTRIBUTING EDITOR Jonathan Hickey

DESIGNER Carter Design, Inc., Denver, Colorado

SPECIAL THANKS TO
Yolanda Blake, Tanya Cochran, Raschelle Casebier, Martin Fancher

Published by AdventHealth
900 Hope Way | Altamonte Springs, FL 32714

For additional copies or volume discounts, please contact AdventHealth at 833-854-8324

CREATIONLife.com

CONTENTS

 LIFE APPLICATION
Personal reflections for your own life

 FOCAL POINT
Things to consider

 IN YOUR OWN WORDS
Apply to your own life

 SMALL GROUP DISCUSSION QUESTIONS
Thoughts to encourage engagement and discussion

 CHECK IT OUT
Evaluate for yourself

 REMEMBER THIS
Ways to embrace life

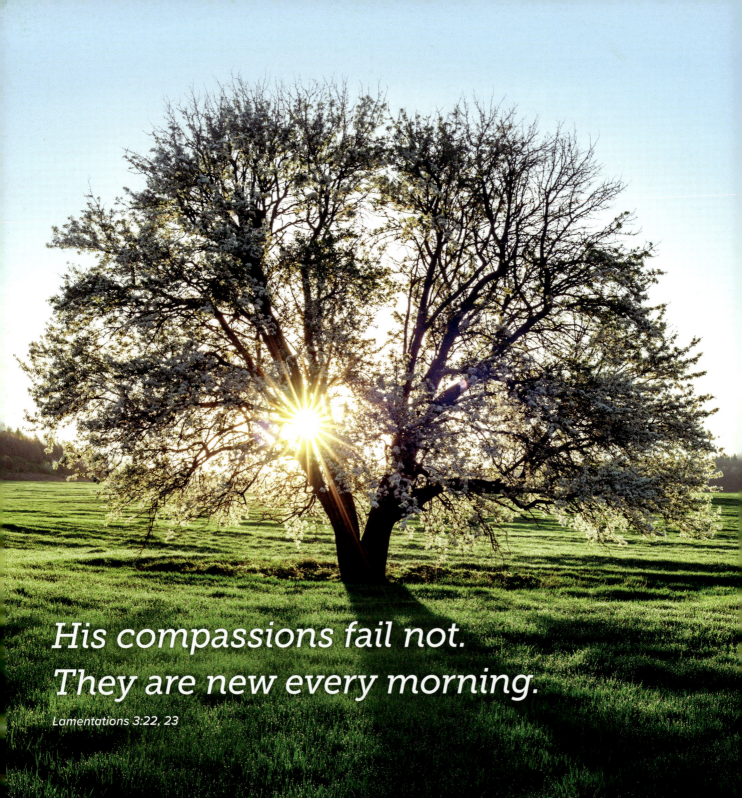

His compassions fail not.
They are new every morning.

Lamentations 3:22, 23

INTRODUCTION

"In the beginning God..."

The quest to discover who we are and where we came from is a journey that has continued for thousands of years. Each successive generation has at some point come face-to-face with these amazing words: "In the beginning God." Just four words into the library we call the Bible, we encounter the biggest idea in the universe: God exists. The Creator of everything desires a friendship with us... with you. Maybe it seems overwhelming or too good to be true, but laying all of that aside for a moment, how do you honestly feel about God?

Where I Am *(Place a mark on the line to show what you're feeling right now.)*

I'm sure "God"
doesn't exist.

I know God exists and is
personally interested in me.

Regardless of where you consider yourself on the spectrum, chances are you are here because you are looking for something — or feel that something is looking for you. Maybe you've come to this place hoping to find answers to difficult questions. Maybe you long to add a spiritual component to your life. It might be that you're not sure if you even believe in God, but can't help wondering why you are on earth.

Perhaps CREATION Life was your first meaningful contact with the Bible. And as your life was radically changed by the eight universal principles for living life to the fullest, you started wondering how the Bible might improve marriage, career and your relationships. So let's take that step together now as we begin our CREATION Life Bible Exploration journey.

WHY THE BIBLE?

The Bible has long held a revered and respected place in literature. Even today, it is the number one best-selling book of all time. There is no other book quite like it. Inside its covers are 66 books that contain history, poetry, prayers, prophecies, memoirs and letters. At least 38 authors and styles of writing appear in three languages.

The Old Testament (OT), composed between 1500 B.C. and 400 B.C., contains more than 300 prophecies about the coming of the Messiah. This unique individual was sent to save His people from their sins and make a way for God and humanity to be together forever. What is truly remarkable is that Jesus of Nazareth fulfilled every prophecy made centuries prior, from the time and place of His birth to the details of His sacrificial death on the cross. The odds of this happening are beyond calculation.

The books of the New Testament (NT) were written between A.D. 50 and A.D. 100, and feature the best ancient manuscript evidence in the world; 24,633 ancient manuscripts of the New Testament exist — more than the next 20 pieces of classical literature combined. Compare that number to Homer's *Iliad*, (the second most-preserved book after the New Testament), which has only 643 extant copies and you'll begin to see how amazing the Bible's preservation has been.

In 2 Timothy 3:16, the Apostle Paul writes, "All Scripture is given by inspiration of God." This means human authors didn't write the Bible alone. God inspired them. He poured His love and thoughts deeply into their minds so that His truth might flow through their words. You can trust the Bible to be God's good news.

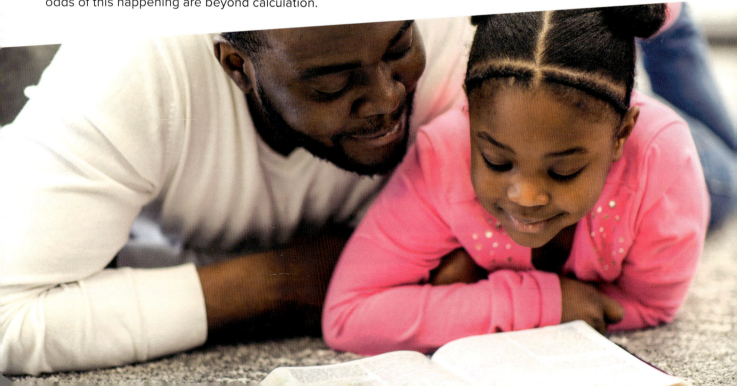

A LOVE STORY

God loves stories and the Bible is the greatest story of all. It's full of action, adventure, suspense and plenty of surprises. Most of all, it's a story about love, how God loved the world so much that He gave His Son, so that whoever believes in Him will not perish but have eternal life (John 3:16). Some have called the Bible "God's Love Letter to You," except that this letter is 30,000 sentences long. Reading and deciphering this letter can feel like a difficult challenge. But in Scripture, God gives a promise to those who seek Him.

And you will seek Me and find Me, when you search for Me with all your heart. I will be found by you, says the Lord.   Jeremiah 29:13,14

God is not hiding. In fact, He longs for you to discover the wondrous things waiting for you in the Bible. Be encouraged and keep reading.

In this special CREATION Life series, the Bible is the foundation for each of our eight studies. But this is more than a Bible study because our aim is to apply Bible principles to our lives.

A father was camping with his young son, and under the soft glow of the moon they hiked along a path through the pine trees. The father held a flashlight to illuminate the way. After a few minutes, the son begged his father to let him hold the flashlight for himself. The father agreed, but upon receiving it the boy immediately pointed the light directly into his own eyes. He was so blinded that he wandered off the path and bumped his head on a low-hanging tree branch. As the father helped his son to his feet he asked why he hadn't kept the light on the path. The embarrassed little boy told his father he thought shining the light in his eyes would "help me see better."

The light of the Bible is designed to illuminate the path of life and light the way for those who are finding their way. But some people aim the Bible directly into their own eyes by amassing great amounts of biblical knowledge or spending much time memorizing texts. They never really apply a working knowledge, or demonstrate a practical understanding of the Bible's principles. They are blinded by their "enlightenment." True enlightenment comes not in learning about God but in encountering God. Many people can talk all day about God (theoretical knowledge), but how much time are they actually spending communicating with God?

CHECK IT OUT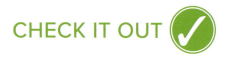

TO ME, THE BIBLE IS:

- ☐ ONE METHOD BY WHICH GOD COMMUNICATES WITH US.
- ☐ MYSTERIOUS AND CONFUSING.
- ☐ GOD'S THOUGHTS IN HUMAN LANGUAGE.
- ☐ SOMETHING ANYBODY CAN SELECTIVELY QUOTE TO "PROVE" ANY POSITION.
- ☐ A TREASURE FIELD FILLED WITH HIDDEN GEMS.
- ☐ TOO MANY "BEGATS" AND "BE IT UNTO THEE FORASMUCH THEREUNTOS."
- ☐ RELEVANT TO MY LIFE TODAY.
- ☐ _____

A kindergartner confessed, "I don't know who God is. We're not up to that yet." As created beings, it's natural for us to struggle with grasping infinity. God is infinite, and to us there will always be a part of God that is a profound mystery.

Yet a mystery is not something we know nothing about; a mystery is something we don't know *everything* about. As with the great Atlantic Ocean, we can know pieces of it. The good news for us is that God has revealed Himself to us in His Word. As we study the Bible, we are always seeking to uncover more truth or evidence. We long to know the One who loves us most in the world, the One who desires for us a full and abundant life.

"These things I have spoken to you, that My joy may remain in you, and that your joy may be full." John 15:11

FOCAL POINT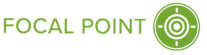

"I have come that _____
                            (YOUR NAME)
may have life, and have it more abundantly." John 10:10

A life with God, while not without its trials, is a life of deep joy that comes from trusting in Him. It's not just our spiritual life God is interested in, but anything that has to do with our well-being.

"And my God shall supply all your needs according to His riches in glory by Christ Jesus." Philippians 4:19

God's desire for us is to find in Him our total wellness, creativity, growth and freedom.

LIST FOUR GIFTS GOD HAS ALREADY GIVEN YOU.

1. ....

2. ....

3. ....

4. ....

God has created the universe based on cause and effect. Simply put, we reap what we sow. Years of poor decision-making will always result in painful consequences regardless of our personal preferences. We can no more escape these results than we can ignore the law of gravity.

By the same token, the universal character laws of love, forgiveness, acceptance, self-discipline and sharing are unchangeable because they too come from God. The more we learn to live a life in accordance to His laws, the more we will have meaningful and lasting success.

"If you know these things, happy are you if you do them." John 13:17

Many people don't pay attention to things like health or relationships until something goes wrong. Tragically, all the money in the world can't always restore it. It is so much better to be proactive by learning from our owner's manual how we were designed to function at our best.

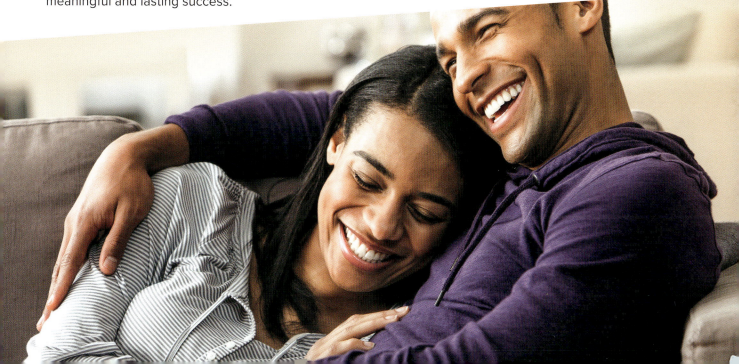

With all of the modern scientific research available today, why should we study the Bible? Perhaps we are drowning in information and thirsting for deep insight. Even with thousands of contemporary books available on practically any subject, we still seek knowledge that goes beyond a "this just in" product line. Possibly we long to combine the latest medical findings with the wisdom of the ages. In addition,

- Living a healthy life helps to lessen the suffering in this world — suffering from broken trust and wounded relationships, addictions and unhealthy habits of sleep, eating and activity.

- CREATION Life brings clarity of mind, which allows us to think and love better.

- CREATION Life reminds us of the Creator's power to re-create His image in us no matter where we are now.

- CREATION Life gives lasting wisdom.

"My people are destroyed for lack of knowledge." Hosea 4:6

Just *knowing* about something isn't enough, though. There's probably not one cigarette smoker who isn't aware that smoking is harmful. But unless you choose to use your knowledge to make changes in your day-to-day life, all the information you have is useless. Jesus' ministry clearly demonstrates His concern for the whole person through teaching (mental), preaching (spiritual), healing (physical), all done "among the people" (social).

"And Jesus went about all Galilee, teaching in their synagogues, preaching the gospel of the kingdom, and healing all kinds of sickness and all kinds of disease among the people." Matthew 4:23

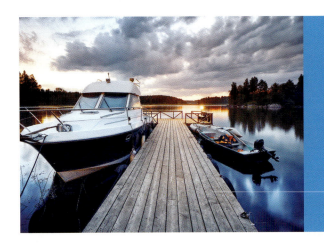

A ship in harbor is safe – but that is not what ships are built for. John A. Shedd

HOW CAN YOU EXPERIENCE OPTIMAL BIBLE STUDY?

For the word of God is living and powerful, and sharper than any two-edged sword, piercing even to the division of soul and spirit, and of joints and marrow, and is a discerner of the thoughts and intents of the heart." Hebrews 4:12

Here are some suggestions for Bible study that millions of people have used with excellent success.

1. OPEN WITH PRAYER

"Open my eyes that I may see wondrous things from Your law." Psalm 119:18

2. STUDY FOR YOURSELF

"Teach me Your way, O Lord; I will walk in Your truth." Psalm 86:11

3. READ REGULARLY

"They received the word with all readiness, and searched the Scriptures daily to find out whether these things were so." Acts 17:11

4. BE TEACHABLE. ASK FOR THE HOLY SPIRIT'S GUIDANCE

"The humble He guides in justice, and the humble He teaches His way." Psalm 25:9

5. TAKE TIME TO CONSIDER EACH CONCEPT AND MEMORIZE A FEW

"Your word I have hidden in my heart, that I might not sin against You." Psalm 119:11

6. SEEK THE TRUTH BEHIND ALL TRUTH

"You search the Scriptures, for in them you think you have eternal life; and these are they which testify of Me. John 5:39

7. APPLY TO YOUR LIFE

"But why do you call Me 'Lord, Lord,' and not do the things which I say? Whoever comes to Me, and hears My sayings and does them, I will show you whom He is like: He is like a man building a house, who dug deep and laid the foundation on the rock. And when the flood arose, the stream beat vehemently against that house, and could not shake it, for it was founded on the rock." Luke 6:46-48

Note: Our compassionate God leads us into truth at a pace we're able to bear.

"I still have many things to say to you, but you cannot bear them now." John 16:12

PRINCIPLES IN LIVING A CREATION LIFE

LOOK FOR THE GOOD, AND CONTINUE FOCUSING ON IT.

Research has found that focusing on the good — the positives — strongly supports a healthy immune system. Focusing on the negatives tends to discourage and bring us down.

God encourages us to concentrate on positive progress. This truly is a key to success.

"The light of the eyes rejoices the heart, and a good report makes the bones healthy." Proverbs 15:30

"Do not be overcome by evil, but overcome evil with good." Romans 12:21

SET S.M.A.R.T. GOALS

Elbert Hubbard observes, "Many people fail in life, not for lack of ability or brains or even courage, but simply because they have never organized their energies around a goal." This is an opportunity for you to set some S.M.A.R.T. goals.

S.M.A.R.T. GOALS ARE...

Specific

Measurable

Attainable

Relevant

Time-bound

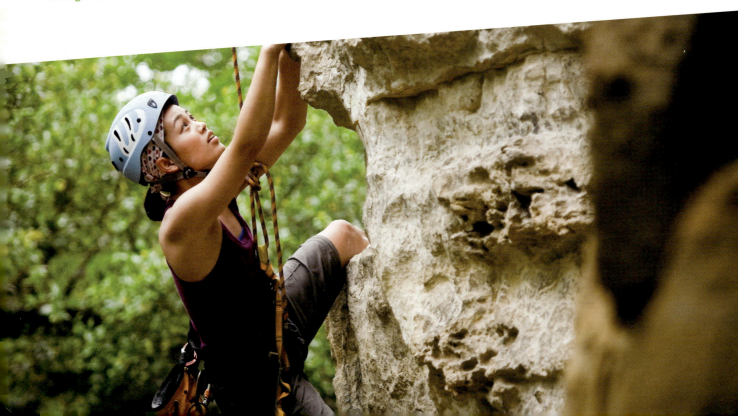

SPECIFIC

A general goal might be, "Get in shape." But a specific goal would begin, "Join the gym and work out three days a week." Make sure your goals are specific enough that you understand what you are working toward.

MEASURABLE

Goals are easier to keep when you can measure your progress. Keep track of your goals in a journal and count down how far you have to go. You'll experience the excitement that comes from all your achievements. Journaling also creates a record that allows you to look back and see just how far you've come.

ATTAINABLE

You can reach almost any goal when you plan your steps wisely and establish a reasonable framework that allows you to carry out those steps. Goals that may have seemed out of reach eventually move closer and become even more attainable.

RELEVANT

Is your goal worth pursuing? Of course you are the only one who can decide that, but don't be afraid to set your sights high. A high goal can be easier to reach than a low one because a low goal exerts low motivational force. Some of the hardest jobs you ever accomplished actually seemed easy in the end because they were a labor of love.

TIME-BOUND

If you want to lose 10 pounds, by what date do you want to lose it? Anchor your goal to a timeline ("by May 15"), and put your unconscious mind into motion to begin working on the goal.

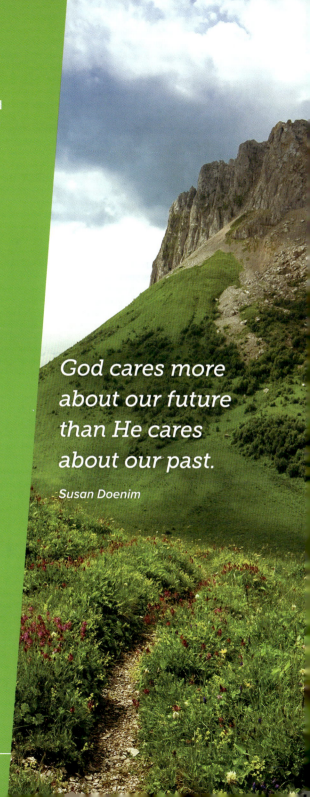

God cares more about our future than He cares about our past.

— Susan Doenim

LIFE APPLICATION

Take a moment to reflect on your goals for your CREATION Life Bible Exploration.

WHAT GOALS DO YOU WANT TO APPLY IN YOUR LIFE?

....

....

....

....

....

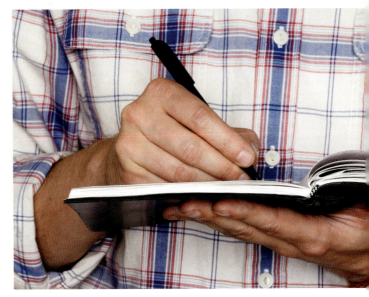

Living a CREATION Life is a process of taking small steps that make a big difference. Unhealthy habits are best "squeezed out." This means that as you add more good things to your life, very little room remains for unhealthy habits.

If you do go back a step or two in pursuing a goal, it's okay because living a CREATION Life is about progress, not perfection. Just keep going and stay true to the vision of who you want to become and press onward. Always take note of any progress and maintain an optimistic attitude. Soon you'll be on your way to completing your S.M.A.R.T. goal!

SMALL GROUP DISCUSSION QUESTIONS

How to Organize a Small Group

Your CREATION Life experience will be enhanced and affirmed when you share it with others. Gather a small group and travel this journey together. At the end, you'll have close, healthy friendships for life.

A NEW BEGINNING

The Almighty Creator, who has the power to turn winter into spring, has the same power to re-create inside of you a new life, with new thoughts and new habits. Whatever your goals, God deeply desires you to succeed and has promised to help you.

Not everything that is faced can be changed, but nothing can be changed until it is faced. *James Baldwin*

How are you feeling right now? *(Place a mark on the line below.)*

Hesitant   **Ready for action**

CREATION Life is about...

• possibilities and potential.

• inspiring you to make progress.

• being all that God created you to be.

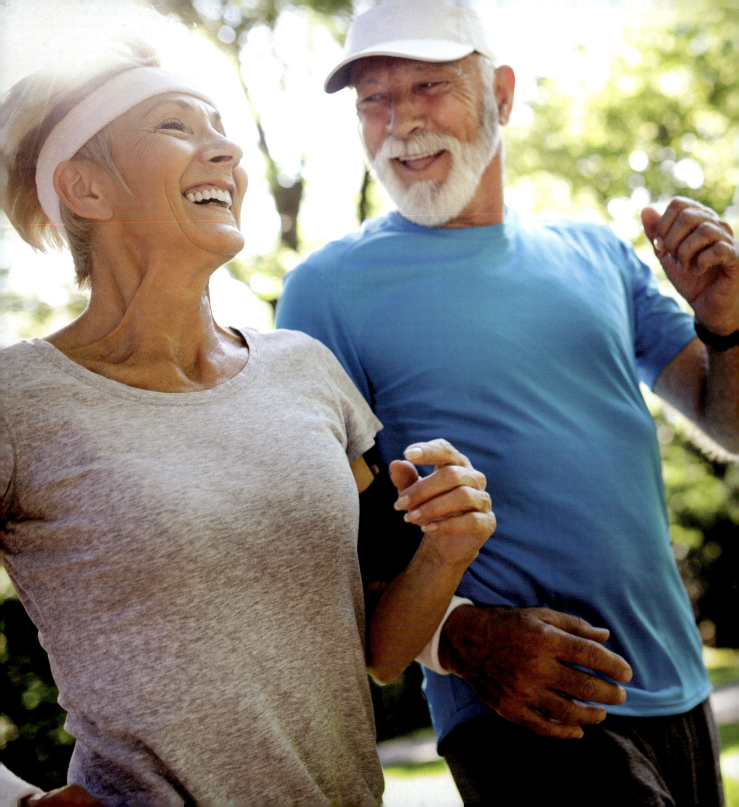

CHOICE

Choose for yourselves this day whom you will serve...
But as for me and my house, we will serve the Lord.

Joshua 24:15

Mavis Lindgren was, in her own words, a "typical grandmother" who, at the age of 62, was living "the usual non-active lifestyle."[1] She was 20 pounds overweight, lacked energy and often fought illness. It was the year she had four bouts of pneumonia that she recognized how badly she needed to change her lifestyle. Mavis attended a lecture that encouraged her to "take responsibility for your own health." Then she made a choice. At first, she was limited in how she could exercise. Because she couldn't run around the block, she began walking in the morning. Gradually she increased the pace.

"I decided to do some fast walking," she remembered. "Then I started a few running steps along the way."

Mavis increased her running until every morning she ran four miles. Her resting pulse dropped from 74 to 54, she lost those 20 pounds and her hemoglobin improved. In addition, she noticed one significant change: "I wasn't sick anymore! Feeling better is such a blessing."

At age 70, Mavis ran her first marathon. During her next race, the Honolulu Marathon, her physician son, Kelvin, joined her for the final two miles. A few hundred feet from the finish, he spotted a physician acquaintance running several paces behind them. "Hey!" he shouted back to the man. "You're not going to let my *mother* beat you, are you?" Spurred on, the desperate man sprinted ahead to the tape.

Between the ages of 70 and 90, "Amazing Mavis" ran 75 marathons, an average of almost four per year. At age 80, clinical tests showed she had the heart and lung efficiency of a normal 22 year old woman.

Mavis Lindgren lived to be 104. Her life continues to inspire people of all ages to take charge of their health and to take the "first step" on the road to change.

THE FIRST STEP

Choice is the first step toward any improvement. Before we can achieve positive, lasting changes in any area of life we must first choose to do so.

In the broadest sense, choice means the ability to evaluate options and select one we prefer — to exercise our willpower. Often we do this unconsciously, but we can never avoid making choices. Even choosing to do nothing exercises our power of choice.

Actually, with very few exceptions (e.g. forgetting something, dreaming or a physical reflex) *everything we do we choose to do.* We choose based on what motivates us — whether it is pleasure and idealism, or unpleasant consequences. We process the cost versus the benefit and then we choose to take action... or not.

"But I didn't want to clean the bathroom," we might say. "I had to do it, so it wasn't my choice." We've all had to do things we didn't want to do but, in the end, we actually chose to do them, usually because the consequences of not doing them were far worse. Consider a child who doesn't want to go to school. Because the consequences of not going are so severe — whether at home or in a future career — she will go. Taking all aspects into account, we choose.

Why does this matter to CREATION Life? Because when we acknowledge the power of choice, we stop feeling like the victim and start taking responsibility for our lives. We may not be able to control everything, but we are always in control of our attitude and how we will respond.

CHECK IT OUT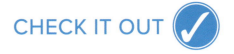

DO YOU AGREE THAT NEARLY EVERYTHING YOU DO IS WHAT YOU CHOOSE TO DO?

YES ☐   **NO** ☐

TOO MANY CHOICES

In his book *The Paradox of Choice: Why More Is Less,* Barry Schwartz probes why being able to choose is healthy, but having too much choice is debilitating. For example, research shows that offering consumers too many flavors of jam (two dozen instead of a half dozen) actually reduces sales. Beyond a certain point, too many options feel paralyzing: more choices means less contentment.

Schwartz describes entering a Gap store and asking for a new pair of blue jeans. The clerk asks if Schwartz wants slim fit, easy fit or relaxed fit; regular or faded; stone-washed or acid-washed; button fly or regular fly. He spends longer in the store than he planned and experiences "no small amount of self-doubt, anxiety and dread." At a local supermarket he finds 85 varieties of crackers, 285 types of cookies, 230 different soups, 120 pasta sauces and 175 kinds of salad dressing.

With so many options available to us, how do we combat the overwhelming sense of having too much choice? Schwartz offers these suggestions:

Enjoy an attitude of gratitude. "With practice," Schwartz says, "we can learn to reflect on how much better things are than they might be." When you feel overwhelmed by multiple choices, first thank God for His blessings.

Value constraint and the power of non-reversible decisions. This applies particularly to life's most important decisions. Getting married and raising a family all involve making crucial choices. No matter what you choose, you're bound to experience doubts later in life. You may meet someone younger, funnier or more caring than your spouse, or wonder what things you could do if you had more free time. But when it comes to your kids or your marriage, this is not about comparison-shopping; instead, decide right now not to allow yourself to go down that path. Choose to focus your energy into making your home life the best it can be.[2]

Recognize you have more important things to do than ponder alternatives. "There are a lot of people walking around, really dissatisfied with their lives, unable to put their fingers on what it is that's so troublesome." Your time is far too valuable to waste it by wondering about what "might have been."

REMEMBER THIS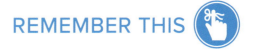

Memorize the following Bible text as an antidote to the tyranny of too many choices:

"I have learned in whatever state I'm in, to be content."
Philippians 4:11

We need to make sure our actions are consistent with our will, our beliefs and what we want for our life. With this gift of choice comes the responsibility to choose wisely.

"God is not the author of confusion but of peace."
1 Corinthians 14:33

NOTE TO READER: In the course of the CREATION Life Bible Exploration you will encounter hundreds of Bible texts. We recommend you **underline** the portions that you especially appreciate. Circle or **Star** the words that apply most to your life.

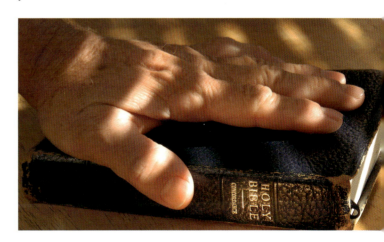

FREEDOM TO CHOOSE

"And the Lord God planted a garden eastward in Eden; and there he put the man whom he had formed. And out of the ground made the Lord God to grow every tree that is pleasant to the sight, and good for food; the tree of life also in the midst of the garden, and the tree of knowledge of good and evil."
Genesis 2:8, 9

"And the Lord God commanded the man, saying, 'Of every tree of the garden you may freely eat; but of the tree of the knowledge of good and evil you shall not eat, for in the day that you eat of it you shall surely die.'" Genesis 2:16, 17

Starting in Eden, God gave humanity the freedom to choose. This gracious gift is emphasized throughout the Bible.

"Stand fast therefore in the liberty by which Christ has set us free, and do not be entangled again with a yoke of bondage." Galatians 5:1

Freedom is sacred to God. He will not force us to be gentle, unselfish, kind or to love Him. God knows love cannot be forced.

This means while God is Sovereign over the entire universe, He has made us sovereign over our own will and our choices. What a wonderful opportunity to cooperate with the One who loves us and longs to truly set us free.

This Bible exploration is not intended to give you merely a list of things you should do or not do. We offer you information that will allow you to make informed decisions.

It is helpful to consider God's example here. In the Garden of Eden He gave humanity the liberty of choice. Throughout His earthly ministry, Jesus maintained a position of respect for the right of every human to choose to follow Him.

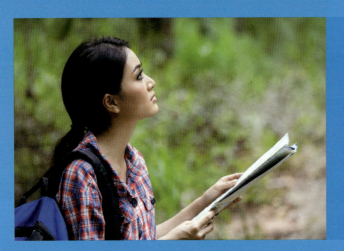

By the choices and acts of our lives, we create the person that we are.

Kenneth Patton

LIFE APPLICATION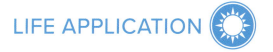

If an all-knowing God does not force His will on us, who are we to think we have the right to coerce others? Also, if freedom is sacred to God, how sacred is freedom to us? Do we stand up for people on the margins of life — those who have no voice or are unable to stand for themselves?

Take a few moments to think about what freedom means to you personally. Which of the famous four freedoms have you been granted?

- Freedom of speech and expression

- Freedom of worship

- Freedom to live healthy lives

- Freedom from fear

IN WHAT WAYS ARE YOU STANDING UP FOR THE FREEDOMS OF OTHERS?

....

....

....

....

....

....

....

....

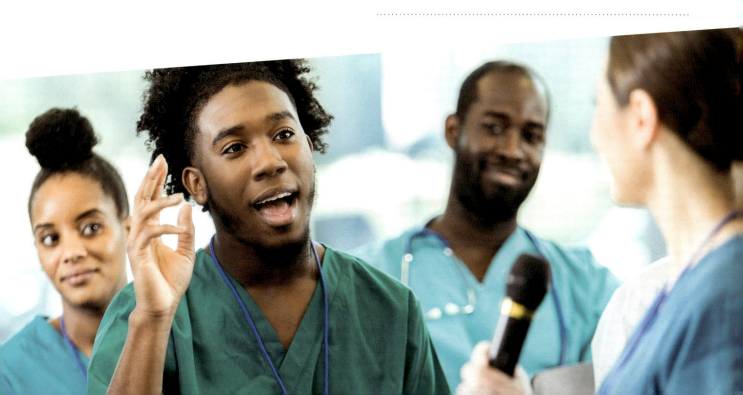

SCRAMBLED EGGS OR OMELETS?

Researchers conducted a study at Shady Grove nursing home on the amount of control the elderly residents had over their daily lives. The participants were divided by floors and closely monitored.

To the first-floor residents, the nursing home director gave this speech: "I'd like you to know about all the things that you can do for yourself here at Shady Grove. There are omelets or scrambled eggs for breakfast, but you have to choose which you want the night before. There are movies on Wednesday or Thursday night, so sign up in advance. Here are some plants; pick one out and take it to your room — but you have to water it yourself."

However, the director gave the second floor residents this speech: "I want you to know about what we can do for you here at Shady Grove. There are omelets or scrambled eggs for breakfast. We make omelets on Monday, Wednesday and Friday, and scrambled eggs on the other days. Movies are on Wednesday and Thursday night. On Thursday nights residents from the left quarter go, Wednesday nights the right quarter goes. Here are some plants for your rooms. The nurse will pick one out for you and she will take care of it."

Each floor received the same things, but the second-floor residents had no choice or control over them. Eighteen months later, the researchers returned to the nursing home. They found that the first-floor residents were more active. Researchers also found that fewer members of this group had died. This study strongly indicated that choice and control could save and enrich lives.[3]

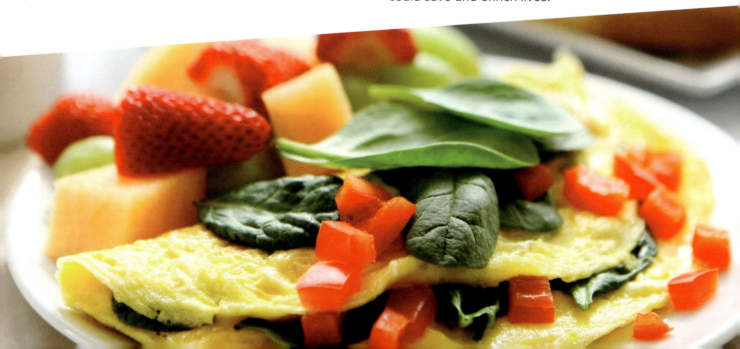

Choose life, that both you and your descendants may live; that you may love the Lord your God, that you may obey His voice, and that you may cling to Him, for He is your life and the length of your days."
Deuteronomy 30:19, 20

"I will instruct you and teach you in the way you should go; I will guide you with My eye."
Psalm 32:8

Of what use is immortality to a man who has not learned to live half an hour?

Ralph Waldo Emerson

IN YOUR OWN WORDS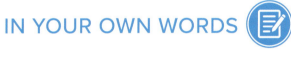

REWRITE THE TWO PREVIOUS TEXTS AS THEY RELATE TO YOUR LIFE.

....

....

....

....

....

....

....

....

....

HOW IMPORTANT
ARE OUR THOUGHTS?

"For as he thinks in his heart, so is he."
Proverbs 23:7

"He who is faithful in what is least is faithful also in much; and he who is unjust in what is least is unjust also in much." Luke 16:10

Consider a compass that is only one degree off. If you are trying to get from here to the nearest grocery store, that degree may not mislead you. However, if you are traveling from Seattle, Washington to Jacksonville, Florida, you may well end up in a different state. So it is with our life's journey; it doesn't take much to veer off course just a fraction of an inch and arrive miles away from our intended destination.

Ask God to help give you wisdom and the power to make the best choices in every situation. Your choices today — even the little ones — will impact your ability to make good choices in the future.

"Prayer is most real," Calvin Miller maintains, "when we refuse to say 'Amen.' We most love heaven when we will not end our conversation quickly."

Listen to Jesus speaking some of the most beautifully assuring words:

"My sheep hear My voice, and I know them, and they follow Me. And I give them eternal life, and they shall never perish; neither shall anyone snatch them out of My hand." John 10:27, 28

Choose your **THOUGHTS**;
they become your words.

Choose your **WORDS**;
they become your actions.

Choose your **ACTIONS**;
they become your habits.

Choose your **HABITS**;
they become your character.

Choose your **CHARACTER**;
it becomes your destiny.

Choose your **DESTINY**;
it becomes your life today and forever.

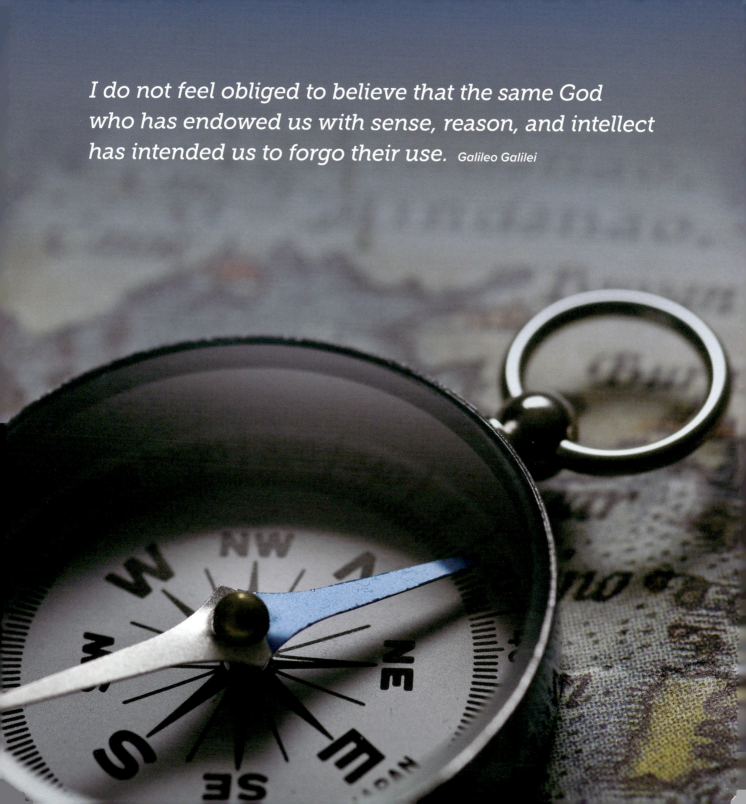

I do not feel obliged to believe that the same God who has endowed us with sense, reason, and intellect has intended us to forgo their use. Galileo Galilei

FOCAL POINT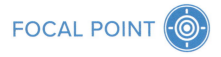

Throughout each day, we can be asking God, "What would you have me do?" Then, *listen* to God's Spirit whispering. This requires *practice*. It requires being still and listening for God's impulse to bring something or someone to mind. Try it now on this calendar page.

God, what would You have me do today?

DATE: **GOD'S PLAN FOR ME TODAY:**

....

....

....

....

....

....

....

....

....

....

....

To Do List:

"Each morning consecrate yourself to God for that day," suggests Ellen White. "Surrender all your plans to Him, to be carried out or given up as His providence shall indicate. Thus day by day you may be giving your life into the hands of God, and thus your life will be molded more and more after the life of Christ."

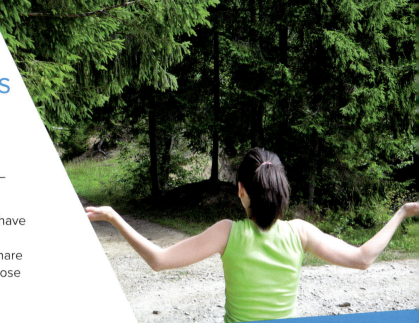

MAKING HEALTHY CHOICES

"I have come that they may have life."
John 10:10

The Greek word for "life" in this passage is ZOË –
"life as God has it."

Take a moment to contemplate the life you now have
and compare it with ZOË — God's life. This
is CREATION Life — a journey that He longs to share
with you. Exercise your power of choice and choose
the ZOË life.

In this CREATION Life Bible Exploration you will discover God's wisdom on how to:

Choose to Rest peacefully and enjoy "nature's sweet restorer."

Choose an Environment you will thrive in.

Choose an Activity for mental and physical growth and strength.

Choose to Trust in God — trust in His power, wisdom and care.

Choose to connect through Interpersonal Relationships.

Choose to form an Outlook on life that reflects your Creator's love.

Choose to enjoy God's bounty by eating the Nutrition of Eden.

"Remove from me the way of lying...
I have chosen the way of truth."
Psalm 119:29, 30

Choosing a life of authenticity isn't easy. When lying appears to be an acceptable approach to life, our spiritual compass will be continually spinning. We must make a strong commitment to total honesty or our integrity will soon disintegrate.

The following poem by Stephen Crane, published in 1899, points out the difficult path of a commitment to truth.

The path to truth is never an easy choice but it's the only path that will bring lasting peace and contentment. We don't need to spend our lives trying to remember which "story" we told. We live as honest and forthright individuals.

THE WAYFARER

The wayfarer,
Perceiving the pathway to truth,
Was struck with astonishment.
It was thickly grown with weeds.
"Ha," he said,
"I see that none has passed here
In a long time."
Later he saw that each weed
Was a singular knife.
"Well," he mumbled at last,
"Doubtless there are other roads."

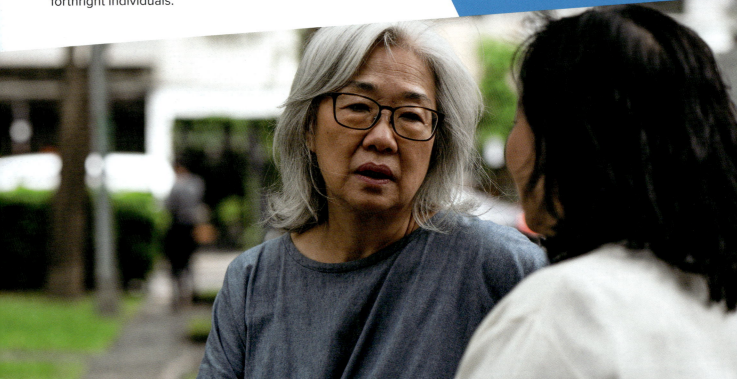

CHOICE OF INTEGRITY

In *Which Jesus? Choosing Between Love and Power*, Tony Campolo writes of a choice for courageous love that conquered the most oppressive evil.

It is the story of Metropolitan Kyril, leader of the Orthodox Church in Bulgaria during World War II. When the Nazis came for the Jews, forcing them into boxcars at the train station in Sophia, Bulgaria, Metropolitan Kyril made a heroic and dangerous choice.

> As the panic-stricken Jews, many sobbing hysterically, awaited their fate, a strange image appeared out of the drizzly, misty night. It was Metropolitan Kyril. He was a tall man to start with, but the miter an Orthodox prelate wears on his head made him look like a giant. His flowing white beard hung down over his black robe, and it is said that his gait was such that the couple hundred men who followed him had to hustle hard to keep up with him.
>
> As he approached the entrance of the barbed-wire enclosure, the SS guards raised their machine guns and told him, 'Father, you cannot go in there!' Metropolitan Kyril defiantly laughed at them, brushed aside the guns and went into the midst of the Jewish prisoners. The apparently doomed Jews gathered around him, wondering what a leader of the Christian community would have to say to them at this desperate time. With arms upraised, Metropolitan Kyril recited one verse of Scripture from the book of Ruth. He helped to change the destiny of a nation as he shouted, 'Wherever you go, I will go — your people will be my people! Your God will be my God!'
>
> With these words, the frightened Jews were suddenly turned into an emboldened mob. They cheered their Christian friend. The Christians on the outside of the barbed wire enclosures cheered with them, and they became one in the Spirit. Responding to the noise at the train station, the townspeople came out of their houses and joined the crowd.
>
> The SS troops, surveying the scene, decided that discretion was the better part of valor. They boarded the train without their captives and left the town. What further evidence do we need to make the case that God's love can provide the motivation for history-changing action?

Where I Am *(Place a mark on the line to show what you're feeling right now.)*

I've made no commitment
to honesty.

I stand for truth
no matter what.

WHAT CAN WE LEARN FROM EXAMPLES OF CHOICE FOUND IN THE BIBLE?

Adam and Eve's tragic choice

"Now the serpent was more cunning than any beast of the field which the Lord God had made. And he said to the woman, 'Has God indeed said, "You shall not eat of every tree of the garden?"'

And the woman said to the serpent, 'We may eat the fruit of the trees of the garden; but of the fruit of the tree which is in the midst of the garden, God has said, "You shall not eat it, nor shall you touch it, lest you die."'

Then the serpent said to the woman, "You will not surely die knowing good and evil.' For God knows that in the day you eat of it your eyes will be opened, and you will be like God, knowing good and evil."

So when the woman saw that the tree was good for food, that it was pleasant to the eyes, and a tree desirable to make one wise, she took of its fruit and ate. She also gave to her husband with her, and he ate.

Then the eyes of both of them were opened, and they knew that they were naked; and they sewed fig leaves together and made themselves coverings."
Genesis 3:1-7

Though they were created perfectly and lived in a perfect environment, Adam and Eve chose to disobey. Their sin has since plagued our world and affected every living thing.

God's response to Adam and Eve's choice — Jesus

"All we like sheep have gone astray; we have turned, every one, to his own way; and the Lord has laid on Him the iniquity of us all. He was oppressed and He was afflicted, yet He opened not His mouth; He was led as a lamb to the slaughter, and as a sheep before its shearers is silent, so He opened not His mouth. He was taken from prison and from judgment, and who will declare His generation? For He was cut off from the land of the living; for the transgressions of My people He was stricken. And they made His grave with the wicked — but with the rich at His death, because He had done no violence, nor was any deceit in His mouth." Isaiah 53:6-9

Jesus chose to come to this earth and give His life for us. Amazing love! It was because of His choice that we can enjoy eternal life, beginning now.

Joseph chose to follow God even after he was sold into slavery.

"Now Joseph had been taken down to Egypt. And Potiphar, an officer of Pharaoh, captain of the guard, an Egyptian, bought him from the Ishmaelites who had taken him down there. The Lord was with Joseph, and he was a successful man; and he was in the house of his master the Egyptian. And his master saw that the Lord was with him and that the Lord made all he did to prosper in his hand. So Joseph found favor in his sight, and served him. Then he made him overseer of his house, and all that he had he put under his authority.

So it was, from the time that he had made him overseer of his house and all that he had, that the Lord blessed the Egyptian's house for Joseph's sake; and the blessing of the Lord was on all that he had in the house and in the field." Genesis 39:1-5

Joseph could have easily grown resentful due to the abuse he suffered at the hands of his brothers, but he chose to stay faithful to the God of his father and to live with integrity. God used Joseph to bless countless people and save them from famine.

Ten thousand difficulties do not make one doubt.

John Henry Newman

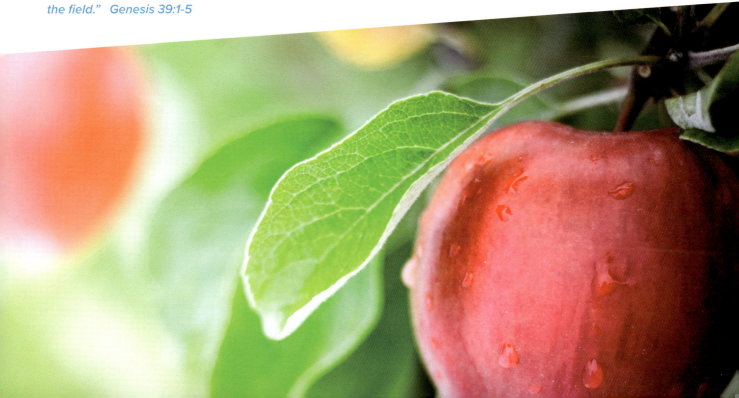

John the Baptist had to make a choice about recognition and power.

"There arose a dispute between some of John's disciples and the Jews about purification.

And they came to John and said to him, 'Rabbi, He who was with you beyond the Jordan, to whom you have testified — behold, He is baptizing, and all are coming to Him!'

John answered and said, 'A man can receive nothing unless it has been given to him from heaven.'

'You yourselves bear me witness, that I said, "I am not the Christ," but "I have been sent before Him."'

'He who has the bride is the bridegroom; but the friend of the bridegroom, who stands and hears him, rejoices greatly because of the bridegroom's voice. Therefore this joy of mine is fulfilled.'

'He must increase, but I must decrease.'"
John 3:25-30

John was sent to prepare hearts for the coming of Jesus. Once Jesus arrived, John lost many of his followers, but he chose to decrease his position and influence, knowing that the people must follow the Good Shepherd.

There are many other Bible characters whose choices made a great impact.

- Abraham, who chose to trust God and leave his country

- Esther, the brave queen

- David, the boy who fought the giant through the power of God

- Stephen, the martyr who stood resolutely for God

The library of the Bible contains inspiring stories of how individuals chose to obey God and follow His plans, and how their devotion resulted in great blessings. May we each think about our choices not only how they impact us personally, but also how our choices impact those whom we love.

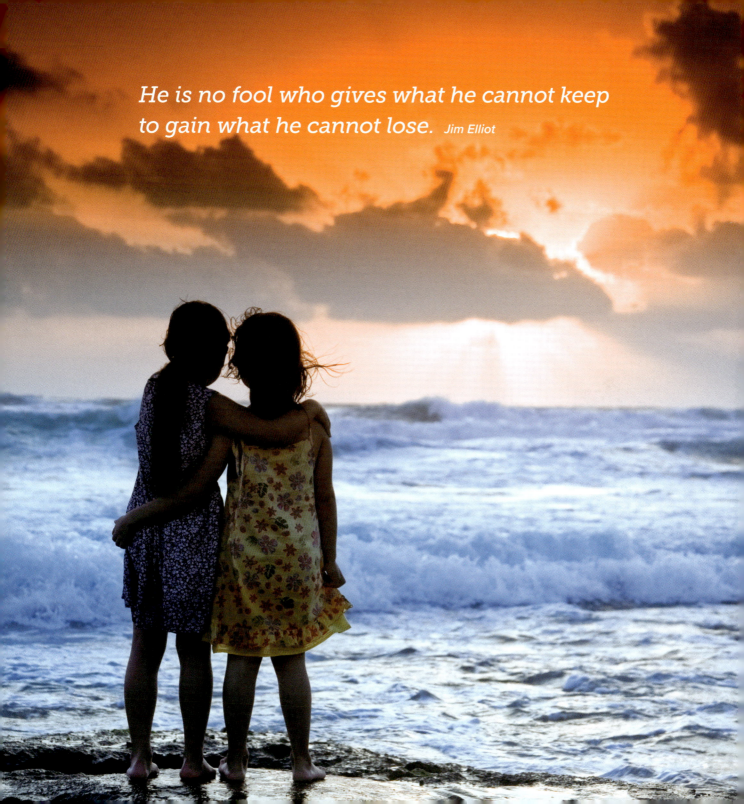

He is no fool who gives what he cannot keep to gain what he cannot lose. *Jim Elliot*

IN YOUR OWN WORDS

LIST FOUR TIMES WHEN YOU FOLLOWED GOD (EVEN IF YOU DIDN'T KNOW IT AT THE TIME) AND WERE BLESSED AS A RESULT.

1. ....

....

2. ....

....

3. ....

....

4. ....

....

CHOICE BENEFITS

"Finally, brothers [and sisters], whatever is true, whatever is noble, whatever is right, whatever is pure, whatever is lovely, whatever is admirable — if anything is excellent or praiseworthy — think about such things." Philippians 4:8

When we fill our lives with the good, beautiful and the lovely, we don't have time to spend on the worthless, meaningless and negative aspects of life. If we can forgive, let go of our hurts and focus on the good attributes of others. Then we can enjoy deeper and more loving relationships. This focus helps us to fill our plates with good food, to fill our nights with peaceful sleep and to surround ourselves with environments that are refreshing and healing. Choosing a positive focus ignites our desire to fulfill our dreams and live purposefully.

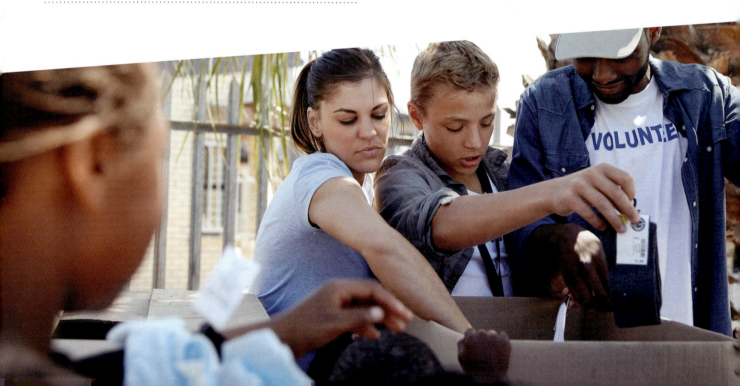

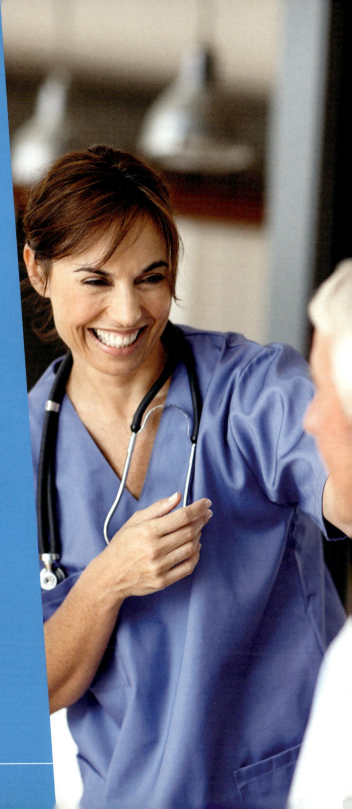

OCCUPATIONAL WELLNESS

Our chosen vocation greatly impacts our health. Do we enjoy our work or do we merely endure it? Is work a constant challenge or constant joy? Work is often a major stressor we face every day.

It's been researched that those who suffer the worst on-the-job stress are people who exercise little control over their jobs. They feel as if they are caught in the middle. This includes cashiers, secretaries, air traffic controllers and assembly line workers. Their ability to make choices increases or reduces their level of harmful stress.

God wants us to be happy, but how can work bring us happiness?

"When you eat the labor of your hands, You shall be happy, and it shall be well with you." Psalm 128:2

"So I perceived that nothing is better than that a man should rejoice in his own works, for that is his heritage." Ecclesiastes 3:22

Most middle-class Americans tend to worship their work, work at their play, and play at their worship. Gordon Dahl

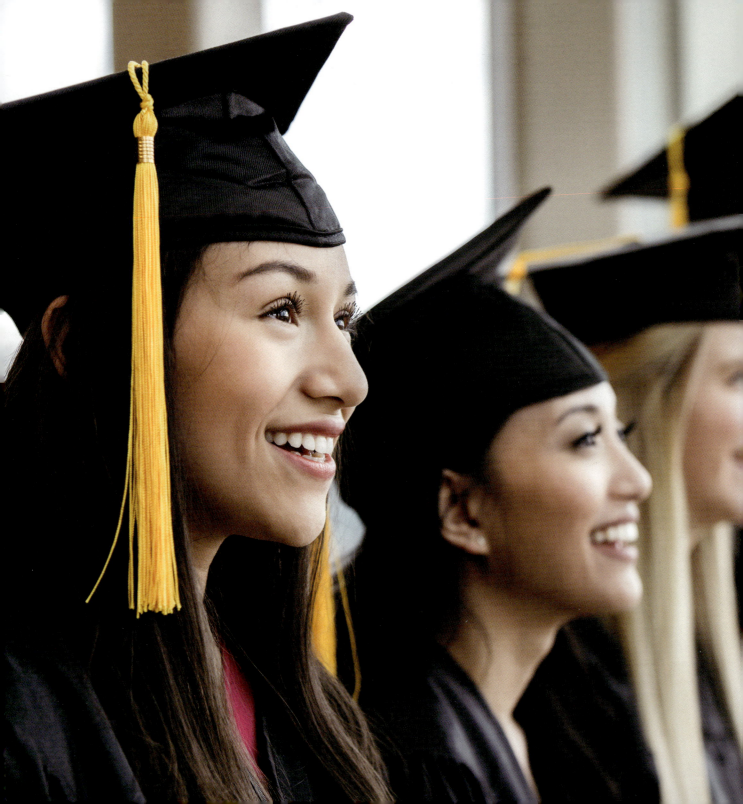

Sometimes God encourages us to do things we are unfamiliar with or have not done before. But whatever God calls you to do, He will equip you with the skills you need. For instance, God spoke to Moses about the value of artists in building the tabernacle:

"'See, I have called by name Bezalel the son of Uri, the son of Hur, of the tribe of Judah. And I have filled him with the Spirit of God, in wisdom, in understanding, in knowledge, and in all manner of workmanship, to design artistic works, to work in gold, in silver, in bronze, in cutting jewels for setting, in carving wood, and to work in all manner of workmanship.'"
Exodus 31:2-5

Are you currently happy at your job? If not, can you think of other skills that God has given you that might bring you more satisfaction and fulfillment? Are you willing to go back to school so that you can be in a career you have a passion for?

> *The one sign of maturity is doing what you have to do when you don't feel like doing it.*
>
> *Chris Blake*

LIFE APPLICATION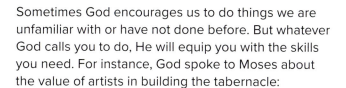

In what ways can you find more fulfillment and meaning in your work? Is there some community service or skill set you can offer that can fill your life with greater purpose?

WRITE A FEW IDEAS HERE:

....

....

....

....

....

....

....

How can you get the most from your work even if you are stressed by it? Take it to a higher level — do it for God.

"And whatever you do, do it heartily, as to the Lord and not to men."
Colossians 3:23

If we are feeling pressured at work and are having a hard time with our co-workers, then a great way to "rise above" these challenges is to choose to work for God. God has always been our real boss and He expects us to do excellent work, no matter how we are being treated or valued. God is also the One who helps us succeed.

WHO COOPERATES AND BLESSES US IN OUR WORK?

"I planted, Apollos watered, but God gave the increase. So then neither he who plants is anything, nor he who waters, but God who gives the increase receive a reward." **1 Corinthians 3:6, 7**

"Unless the Lord builds the house, they labor in vain who build it; unless the Lord guards the city, the watchman stays awake in vain." **Psalm 127:1**

"Lord, You will establish peace for us, for You have also done all our works in us." **Isaiah 26:12**

It's good to feel the full blessing and cooperation of God as we go about our daily endeavors. God also wants us to be active participants in His work.

"I have seen the God-given task with which the sons of men are to be occupied. He has made everything beautiful in its time. Also He has put eternity in their hearts, except that no one can find out the work that God does from beginning to end. I know that nothing is better for them than to rejoice, and to do good in their lives, and also that every man should eat and drink and enjoy the good of all his labor — it is the gift of God." **Ecclesiastes 3:9-13**

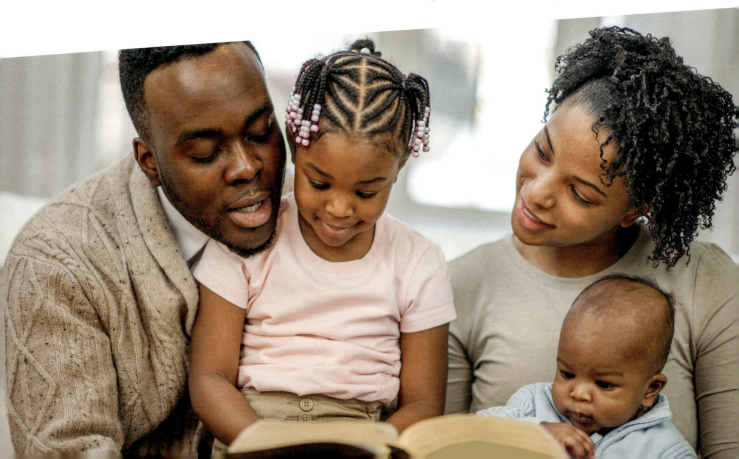

BIBLE THOUGHTS ON LAZINESS

"The soul of a lazy man desires, and has nothing; but the soul of the diligent shall be made rich."
Proverbs 13:4

"In all labor there is profit, but idle chatter leads only to poverty." Proverbs 14:23

God understands our natural inclination toward laziness. That's why the book of Proverbs gives us several encouragements to be responsible, proactive and productive.

"He who tills his land will have plenty of bread, but he who follows frivolity will have poverty enough!"
Proverbs 28:19

The Bible warns us about following frivolity — doing something of little value or significance. God has given each day to us as a gift, but we choose how to use it. We can either work at a task that is of value and will benefit those around us, or waste our time with laziness or frivolous activities. It all depends on which we desire most.

"The desire of the lazy man kills him, for his hands refuse to labor. He covets greedily all day long, but the righteous gives and does not spare."
Proverbs 21:25, 26

"The lazy man will not plow because of winter; he will beg during harvest and have nothing."
Proverbs 20:4

God exhorts the lazy to "work harder" and to the workaholic He says, "take it easy." Sadly, it's the sluggard who often relaxes while the frenzied worker increases efforts. The question is, "What do I need to hear?" Is God telling you to "get to work," or is He reminding you to "slow down"?

CHECK IT OUT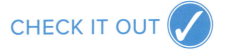

RIGHT NOW, TO ACHIEVE BALANCE AT WORK I NEED TO:

☐ **WORK SMARTER.**

☐ **TAKE A BREAK; BACK OFF.**

☐ **CAP: Communicate, Adapt and Problem-solve.**

☐ **REALLY BEAR DOWN FOR A WHILE.**

☐ **FIND A REJUVENATING OUTLET.**

☐

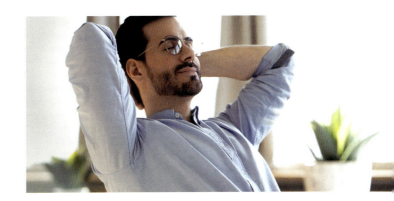

HOW TO GET BEST RESULTS FROM OUR WORK

COMMIT YOUR WORK TO GOD AND ACKNOWLEDGE HIM

"Commit your way to the Lord, trust also in Him, and He shall bring it to pass." Psalm 37:5

"In all your ways acknowledge Him, and He shall direct your paths." Proverbs 3:6

DON'T OVERWORK

"Do not overwork to be rich; because of your own understanding, cease!" Proverbs 23:4

God encourages us to maintain balance in our lives. We should never overwork and strain ourselves in pursuit of riches. When we do we often sacrifice what is most important: our relationship to God and our family.

WORK EFFECTIVELY AND YOU WILL GET GOOD RETURNS

"But this I say: He who sows sparingly will also reap sparingly, and he who sows bountifully will also reap bountifully." 2 Corinthians 9:6

SEEK GOD'S WISDOM TO ENJOY SUCCESS

"Through wisdom a house is built, and by understanding it is established; by knowledge the rooms are filled with all precious and pleasant riches." Proverbs 24:3, 4

Of course we can't stop all problems from developing, but God's wisdom will help us deal with these problems in an effective manner. With His help we may even begin to view our obstacles as opportunities.

WORK IN AN ORDERLY FASHION

"The plans of the diligent lead surely to plenty, but those of everyone who is hasty, surely to poverty." Proverbs 21:5

Think about a project that you are about to work on or are currently working on. Can you prayerfully think of more productive ways to develop this project? Are you using your resources of time and people in the most effective way? Careful, diligent planning leads to success while reckless carelessness causes more trouble and creates a world of new problems. There's a saying in the restaurant business, "You can have it fast, cheap and good, but you can only pick two." Learn to evaluate your work and seek order in all your endeavors.

FINANCIAL WELLNESS

af-flu-en-za n.1. an epidemic of stress, overwork, waste, indebtedness and misplaced priorities caused by dogged pursuit of affluence. 2. an unsustainable addiction to economic growth. 3. the sluggish, heartless, unfulfilled feeling that results from this addiction.

According to the Public Broadcasting System television program "Affluenza," money plays the major role in 90 percent of U.S. divorces. Could our culture of consumerism be to blame? By the age of 20, the average American has seen one million commercials. Americans also carry a total of more than one billion credit cards.

Our financial health is important to God. This is well illustrated by the number of scriptures that speak to financial issues. In his topical scriptural commentary titled, *The Word on Finances*, Larry Burkett discovered more than one thousand references to money in the Bible, second only to the subject of love.

He that is of the opinion money will do everything may well be suspected of doing everything for money.

Benjamin Franklin

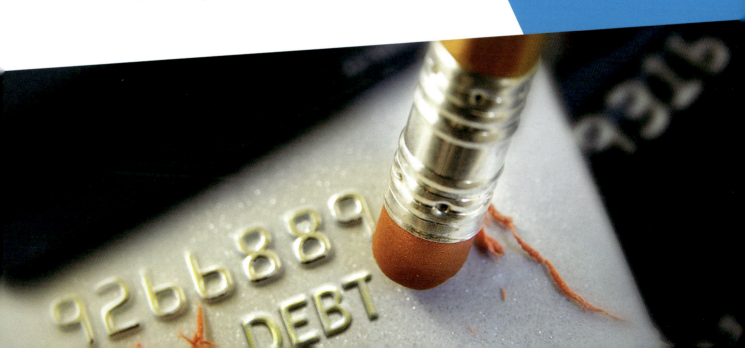

CAN MONEY MANAGEMENT ENHANCE OUR HEALTH?

"Now acquaint yourself with Him, and be at peace; thereby good will come to you."   Job 22:21

"Beloved, I pray that you may prosper in all things and be in health, just as your soul prospers."
3 John 2

When we manage the money God has lent us, we experience improved health in many realms — emotional, spiritual and professional. It's difficult for a person whose finances are in shambles to keep focused on their job, family and friendship with God.

"He who trusts in his riches will fall, but the righteous will flourish like foliage."   Proverbs 11:28

"Remove falsehood and lies far from me; give me neither poverty nor riches — feed me with the food allotted to me; lest I be full and deny You, and say, 'Who is the Lord?' Or lest I be poor and steal, and profane the name of my God."   Proverbs 30:8, 9

Notice the Proverbs 30 request of God: "Give me neither poverty nor riches." What the author is really asking God for is to have his immediate needs met. With an abundance of riches he fears he will forget God and turn away, but with too little he fears disgracing the name of God by stealing. "Just give me what I need — no more, no less."

What do you think? Could you pray that prayer right now?

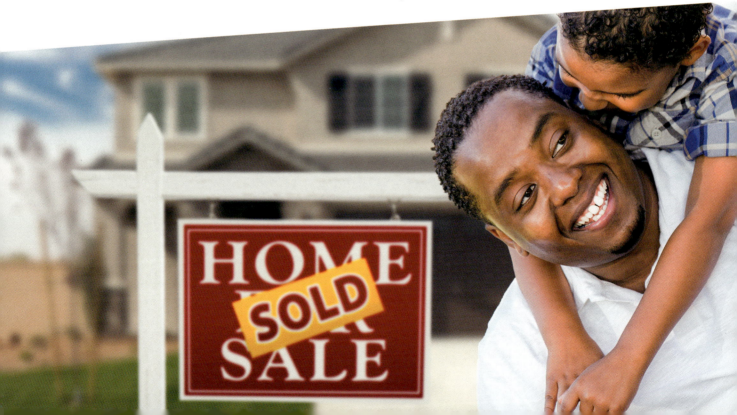

Matthew 13:22 speaks about the "deceitfulness of riches." An improper view of money can produce many problems. Here are just four:

1. The thought that the wealthy are superior to others

2. The belief that gain is godliness

3. The idea that the wealthy are superior in wisdom and judgment to those in poverty

4. The sense that accumulating wealth will bring happiness

Poet E. E. Cummings quipped, "I'm living so far beyond my income that we may almost be said to be living apart." While we may smile at this wordplay, when financial strife hits personally, it really hurts.

"Now godliness with contentment is great gain. For we brought nothing into this world, and it is certain we can carry nothing out. And having food and clothing, with these we shall be content. But those who desire to be rich fall into temptation and a snare, and into many foolish and harmful lusts which drown men in destruction and perdition. For the love of money is a root of all kinds of evil, for which some have strayed from the faith in their greediness, and pierced themselves through with many sorrows."
1 Timothy 6:6-10

> ## *The best way to make your dreams come true is to wake up.* J. M. Power

Notice that money by itself is not the root of evil. It is the *love* of money that is the problem. Money is like electricity — a power that can both heal and kill. We must learn to use this power wisely or else it will have negative effects on our lives.

"Let no debt remain outstanding, except the continuing debt to love one another, for he who loves his fellowman has fulfilled the law." Romans 13:8

Author and radio personality Dave Ramsey points out how we have all seen a child in a toy store screaming, "I want it! I want it! I want it!" This demand frustrates and embarrasses parents and observers alike. Then Dave brings the point home to us "adults." Inside each of us is an I-Want-It Kid. Unless we train that child to live within its means, embarrassment, frustration and shame will come.

We all know people who live within their means and those who don't. Which group do we observe being in financial bondage and which do we see enjoying financial freedom?

WHAT IF WE DO NOT HAVE ENOUGH MONEY?

"Let your conduct be without covetousness; be content with such things as you have. For He Himself has said, 'I will never leave you nor forsake you.'" Hebrews 13:5

"But I am poor and needy; yet the Lord thinks upon me. You are my help and my deliverer; do not delay, O my God." Psalm 40:17

"For He will deliver the needy when he cries, the poor also, and him who has no helper." Psalm 72:12

An ancient parable from India describes a wise woman who found a precious gem in a stream while traveling in the mountains. The next day she met a hungry traveler, so the wise woman shared her food with him. When she opened her bag, the traveler spotted the gem and asked her to give it to him. She gave it without hesitation.

The traveler left, rejoicing. He knew that the stone was valuable enough to provide him security for a lifetime. But a few days later, he returned the gem to the wise woman.

"I've been thinking," he said, "I know how precious the gem is, and I know you know. I bring it back in the hope that you can give me something even more valuable. Give me what you have within you that enabled you to give me the gem."

HELPING AND SHARING

Perhaps you're familiar with Jesus' parable of the Good Samaritan in Luke 10:25–37. This beautiful story is actually a radical prescription for living.

The Old Testament had clearly taught the Jews to "Love your neighbor as yourself," but just exactly who is our neighbor? What determination are we supposed to use? Jesus taught us through the example of the Good Samaritan that anyone in need is our neighbor.

"'If there is among you a poor man of your brethren, within any of the gates in your land which the Lord your God is giving you, you shall not harden your heart nor shut your hand from your poor brother, but you shall open your hand wide to him and willingly lend him sufficient for his need, whatever he needs…. For the poor will never cease from the land; therefore I command you, saying, "You shall open your hand wide to your brother, to your poor and your needy, in your land."' Deuteronomy 15:7, 8, 11

"Then He also said to him who invited Him, 'When you give a dinner or a supper, do not ask your friends, your brothers, your relatives, nor rich neighbors, lest they also invite you back, and you be repaid. But when you give a feast, invite the poor, the maimed, the lame, the blind. And you will be blessed, because they cannot repay you; for you shall be repaid at the resurrection of the just.'" Luke 14:12-14

"The generous soul will be made rich, and he who waters will also be watered himself." Proverbs 11:25

IN YOUR OWN WORDS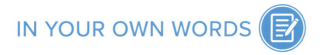

REWRITE THE THREE PREVIOUS TEXTS TO RELATE TO YOUR LIFE.

....

....

....

....

....

....

....

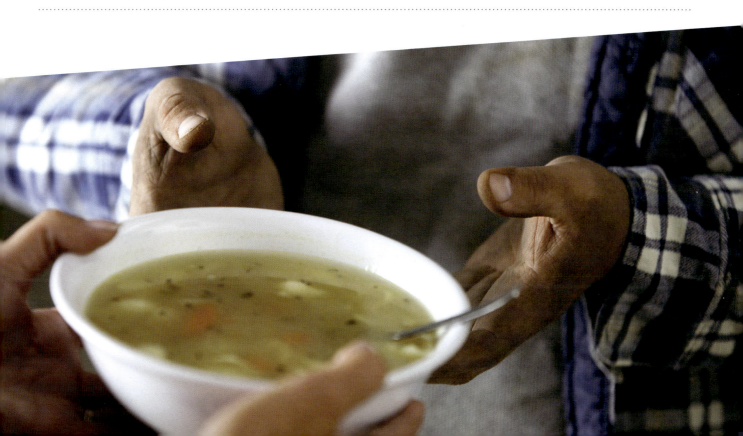

PURSUITS REGARDING WEALTH THAT GOD CONDEMNS

A. BENEFITING ONESELF AT THE EXPENSE OF OTHERS. THIS VIOLATES THE GOLDEN RULE:

"Therefore, whatever you want men to do to you, do also to them, for this is the Law and the Prophets." Matthew 7:12

B. TRUSTING MONEY INSTEAD OF GOD.

"Command those who are rich in this present age not to be haughty, nor to trust in uncertain riches but in the living God, who gives us richly all things to enjoy." Timothy 6:17

"Then Jesus looked around and said to His disciples, 'How hard it is for those who have riches to enter the kingdom of God!' And the disciples were astonished at His words. But Jesus answered again and said to them, 'Children, how hard it is for those who trust in riches to enter the kingdom of God!'" Mark 10:23, 24

Whenever Jesus says something twice, we can be certain He wants us to pay particular attention. Riches will never give us eternal life. Only trust in God can provide that.

Love people and use things; don't love things and use people.

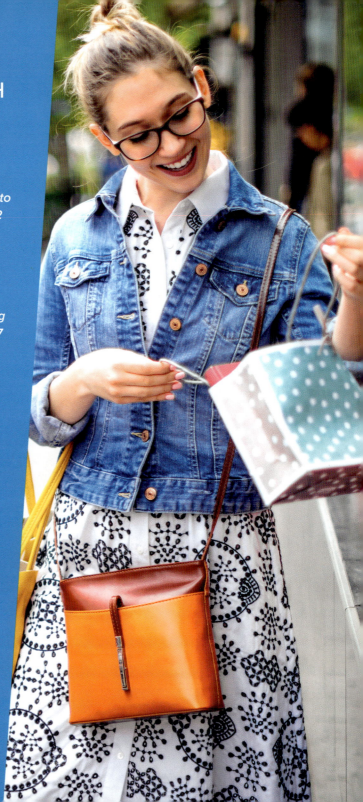

CHECK IT OUT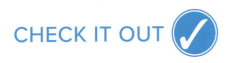

WHAT ARE THE REASONS GOD GAVE US MONEY?

- ☐ MEET OUR NEEDS
- ☐ AS A REWARD FOR OUR GOOD DEEDS
- ☐ BLESS OTHERS
- ☐ HELP US LEARN TO HANDLE BLESSINGS RESPONSIBLY
- ☐ BECAUSE THE PERSON WHO DIES WITH THE MOST TOYS WINS
- ☐ SPREAD HIS LOVE LOCALLY AND WORLDWIDE

LIFE APPLICATION

Take a moment to reflect on this CREATION Life study on choice.

WHAT PRINCIPLES HAVE YOU LEARNED THAT YOU WANT TO APPLY IN YOUR LIFE?

....

....

....

NOW, CREATE A PERSONAL GOAL FOR THE CHOICES IN YOUR LIFE.

....

....

....

Now take a few moments and decide if, at this point in your life, you should act upon the above item or other principles in this section and create two S.M.A.R.T. personal goals. Remember Specific, Measurable, Attainable, Relevant and Time-bound.

Examples of S.M.A.R.T. goals for choice:

My goal is to daily commit to live a life of integrity and love.

My goal is to combat my negative thoughts by memorizing Philippians 4:8 and asking God to help me to choose to focus on the good.

My goal is to sign up for a program (with my spouse, if married) that will help me live within my means.

My goal is to go back to school next fall to be able to work on a new career.

My goal is to do community service at

....

once a month using my God-given skill of

....

MY S.M.A.R.T. GOAL IS TO...

....

1.

....

....

....

2.

....

....

....

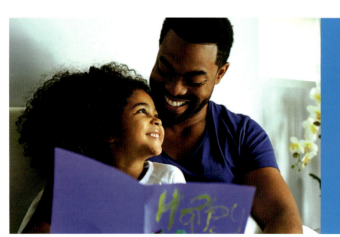

From everyone to whom much is given, much will be required. *Luke 12:48*

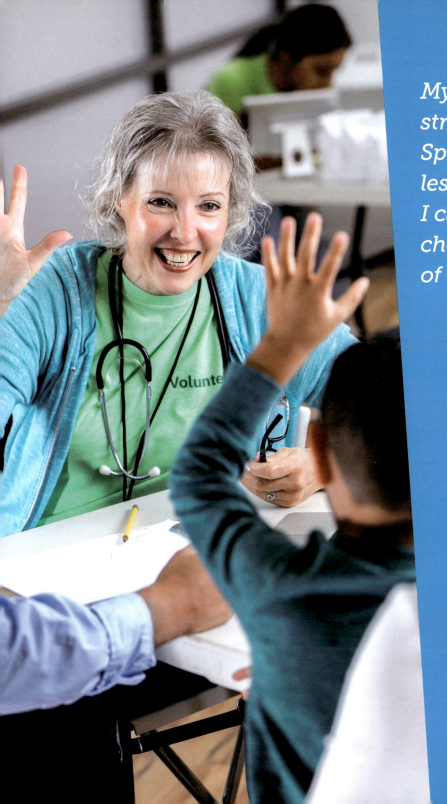

My Prayer: God, please strengthen me with Your Spirit. Help me apply the lessons I have learned so I can enjoy making wise choices every moment of every day.

SMALL GROUP DISCUSSION QUESTIONS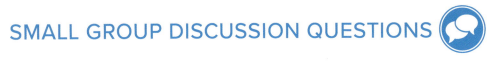

1. **WHAT BIBLE TEXT ON CHOICE IMPACTED YOU MOST?**

....

....

....

....

....

2. **HOW DOES A COMMITMENT TO HONESTY AFFECT ALL CHOICES?**

....

....

....

....

....

3. **A JOKE GOES, "I WONDERED WHY THE BASEBALL KEPT GETTING BIGGER. THEN IT HIT ME." WHICH STORY IN THIS SECTION "HIT" YOU?**

....

....

....

....

....

4. **WHAT INSIGHT ON OCCUPATIONAL HEALTH DID YOU APPRECIATE?**

....

....

....

....

5. **WHAT PRINCIPLE STOOD OUT TO YOU REGARDING FINANCIAL HEALTH?**

....

....

....

....

6. **SHARE A LIFE APPLICATION OF YOURS WITH THE GROUP.**

To lose fat, sleep better, Bible study

....

....

....

7. **SUMMARIZE THREE KEY POINTS OF THIS LESSON.**

Choice, diet, lifestyle

....

....

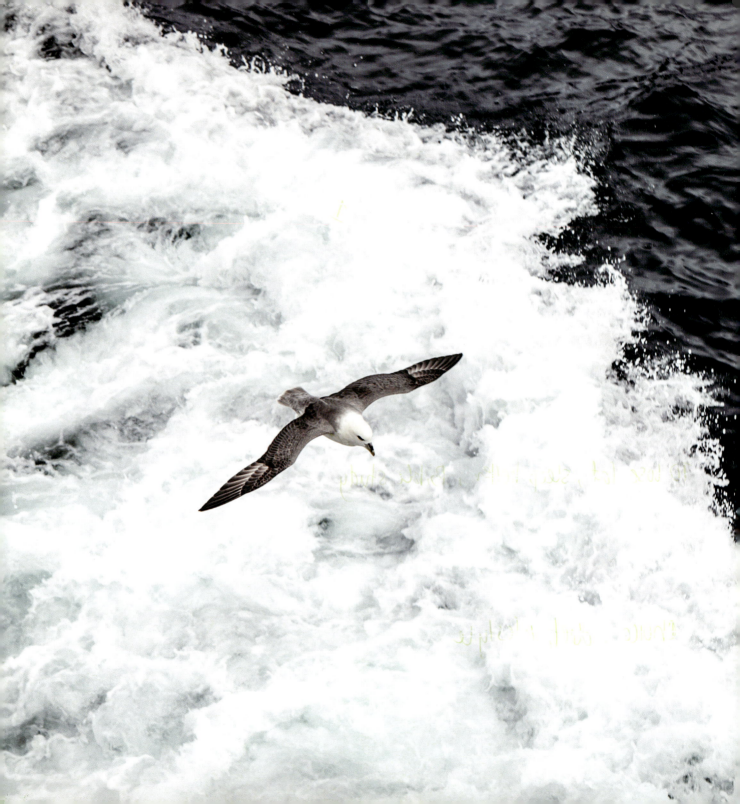

REST

Come to Me, all you who labor and are heavy laden, and I will give you rest. Take My yoke upon you and learn from Me, for I am gentle and lowly in heart, and you will find rest for your souls.

Matthew 11:28, 29

An art contest was once held with the objective to depict peace. Entries poured in, paintings of mist-veiled waterfalls, barefoot lovers strolling along endless sand, sublime sunsets, suckling babies and azure mountain lakes mirroring snow-capped mountains. However, the winner was none of these.

The winning entry depicted a terrific storm at sea. Rain like liquid bullets fell in torrents. Ferocious winds whipped towering waves. Dark, heavy clouds pressed down while lightning stabbed the sky. In the very midst of this turmoil, along the curl of a wave, a single seagull glided serenely.

The gull's progress did not require tranquil surroundings. Its happiness wasn't dependent on circumstances. It carried inner peace.

There is no pillow so soft as a clear conscience.

French Proverb

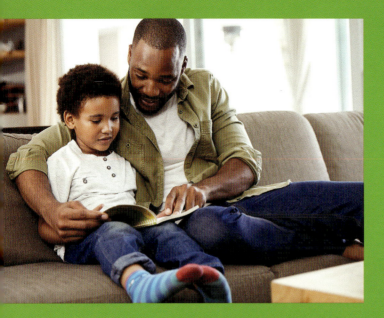

God gave us the gift of nightly rest to calm and rejuvenate us. In Genesis we see God creating the night-and-day pattern as His first act of creation.

"Then God said, 'Let there be light;' and there was light. And God saw the light, that it was good: and God divided the light from the darkness. God called the light Day, and the darkness He called Night. So the evening and the morning were the first day." Genesis 1:3-5

But He didn't stop there. In Genesis 2, God's concluding act of creation was the gift of the Sabbath, a time set apart for rest, reflection and communion with Him.

"Then God blessed the seventh day and sanctified it, because in it He rested from all His work which He had done." Genesis 2:3

Rest is the key to our sanity and survival. While strong research supports the importance of daily rest, both sleeping at night and relaxing during the day, in the Creation story we see the reason: This is truly how God designed us to operate.

This world is full of cares that make us weary. Strained relationships, heavy work loads and financial burdens all take a stressful toll. But whatever our situation, God desires to give us rest.

When we come to Him and follow His ways, He will provide true rest in every sense. Look at Psalm 23 and find how God promises to give rest to His followers.

Where I Am *(Place a mark on the line to show what you're feeling right now.)*

I always feel weary and burdened.

I am well rested and full of energy.

"The Lord is my shepherd; I shall not want [mentally]. He makes me to lie down in green pastures; He leads me beside the still waters [physically]. He restores my soul [spiritually]; He leads me in the paths of righteousness [ethically] for His name's sake. Yea, though I walk through the valley of the shadow of death, I will fear no evil [fearlessly]; for You are with me; Your rod and Your staff, they comfort me [emotionally]. You prepare a table before me in the presence of my enemies [socially]; You anoint my head with oil; my cup runs over [abundantly]. Surely goodness and mercy shall follow me all the days of my life [mercifully]; and I will dwell in the house of the Lord forever [infinitely]."   Psalm 23

My Presence will go with you, and I will give you rest.

Exodus 33:14

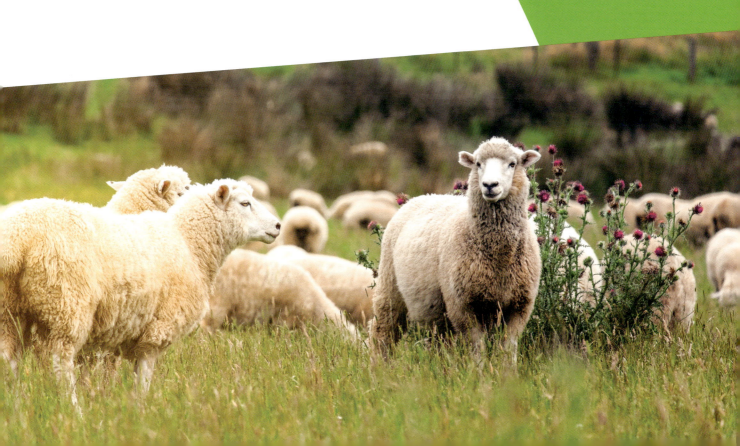

We find true rest by following God's instructions, and there's more. A life devoted to God also promotes our contented happiness.

"Thus says the Lord: 'Stand in the ways and see, and ask for the old paths, where the good way is, and walk in it; then you will find rest for your souls.'"
Jeremiah 6:16

"So God's rest is there for people to enter. But those who formerly heard the Good News failed to enter because they disobeyed God."
Hebrews 4:6

"When you lie down, you will not be afraid; yes, you will lie down and your sleep will be sweet."
Proverbs 3:24

IN YOUR OWN WORDS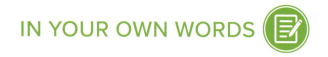

WHAT DO THE PREVIOUS THREE TEXTS SAY ABOUT FINDING REST IN GOD?

....

....

....

....

....

....

....

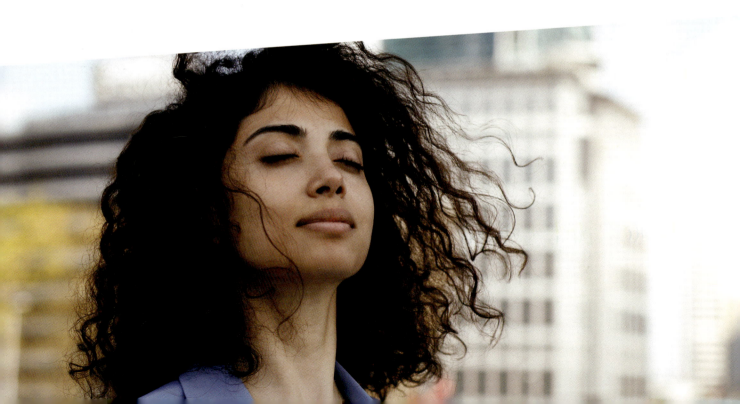

SHALOM

The Hebrew word *shalom* means "peace." This peace is more than just an absence of conflict. *Shalom* is an all-encompassing peace that includes soundness, prosperity and completeness. Jesus came to earth as the Prince of Peace — the Prince of *Shalom* (see Isaiah 9:6) to usher in an era of total peace between God and humanity.

"Peace I leave with you, My peace I give to you; not as the world gives do I give to you. Let not your heart be troubled, neither let it be afraid." John 14:27

As Martin Weber points out, this *shalom* peace is a circle of ever-expanding ripples.

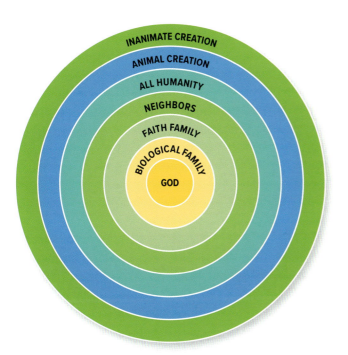

God. Personal peace with God starts with our friendship with our Creator and Redeemer.

Biological family. *Shalom* works to create peace within our family.

Faith family. To those who share our faith yet differ in so many ways, we extend *shalom*.

Neighbors. In the workplace, marketplace, classroom, neighborhood — with those we see and touch — the ripples of *shalom* represent God's love as we consistently seek win-win relationships.

All humanity. Yearning to relieve suffering, we extend *shalom* even to our enemies.

Animal creation. We care for non-human creatures and are reluctant to exploit them.

Inanimate creation. God expects us to be responsible caretakers of the world in anticipation of and practice for the earth made new. We care for the environment and for all created beings.

All of the above was envisioned when Jesus proclaimed literally, "Blessed are the *shalom*-makers."

Blessed are the peacemakers: for they shall be called the children of God.

Matthew 5:9

JESUS IN THE STORM

"On the same day, when evening had come, He said to them, 'Let us cross over to the other side.' Now when they had left the multitude, they took Him along in the boat as He was. And other little boats were also with Him.

And a great windstorm arose, and the waves beat into the boat, so that it was already filling. But He was in the stern, asleep on a pillow. And they awoke Him and said to Him, 'Teacher, do You not care that we are perishing?'

Then He arose and rebuked the wind, and said to the sea, 'Peace, be still!' And the wind ceased and there was a great calm. But He said to them, 'Why are you so fearful? How is it that you have no faith?'

And they feared exceedingly, and said to one another, 'Who can this be, that even the wind and the sea obey Him!'" Mark 4:35-41

Amid the tempests in our lives, God tells us "Peace, be still." He counsels us to simply know that He is God and experience a great calm. Even when events seem to be all wrong, the amazing God of recovery can bring good from them.

Sometimes God calms the storm. Sometimes God lets the storm rage and calms His children.

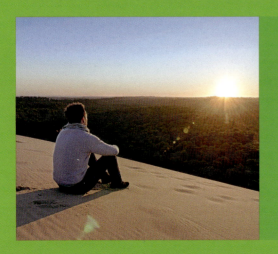

My Prayer: God, help me to be a peacemaker. I desire the true rest and peace that You long to give. Fill me completely with Your calm. May I communicate that shalom to others.

LIFE APPLICATION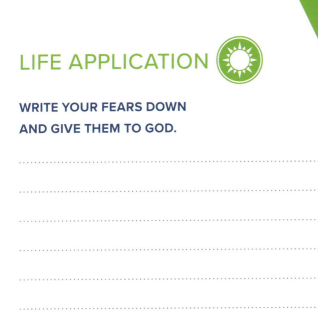

**WRITE YOUR FEARS DOWN
AND GIVE THEM TO GOD.**

....

....

....

....

....

....

....

You will no longer be ruled by fear. Thank Him for your peace.

"These things I have spoken to you, that in Me you may have peace. In the world you will have tribulation; but be of good cheer, I have overcome the world." John 16:33

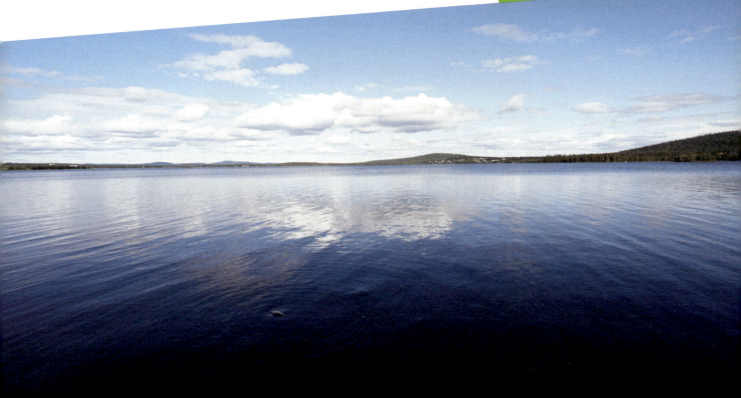

REST FROM GUILT

We are all sinners; we have all done wrong. Perhaps you don't need the Bible to tell you that. In Jesus, you can find forgiveness and experience the peace that this forgiveness brings. Do you desire true rest from the weight of your wrongs and a guilty conscience?

"I, even I, am He who blots out your transgressions, for My own sake, and I will not remember your sins." Isaiah 43:25

"Let it be it known to you therefore, my brothers, that through this Man (Jesus) forgiveness of sins is proclaimed to you." Acts 13:38

"So if the Son sets you free, you will be free indeed." John 8:36

God's forgiveness of our sins helps bring about true rest from guilt. The Bible calls this forgiveness "justification by faith." That means we are not forgiven through any good we have done but only through believing and clinging to God's promises through Jesus. Anyone, no matter their past, can be forgiven because of Jesus. A sinner admits his or her sin, and then claims, by faith, the perfect life of Jesus as their substitute.

God not only forgives their sins, but Jesus' life is credited to them as if it were their own. They then stand justified (made right) before God. It's a wonderful gift of grace.

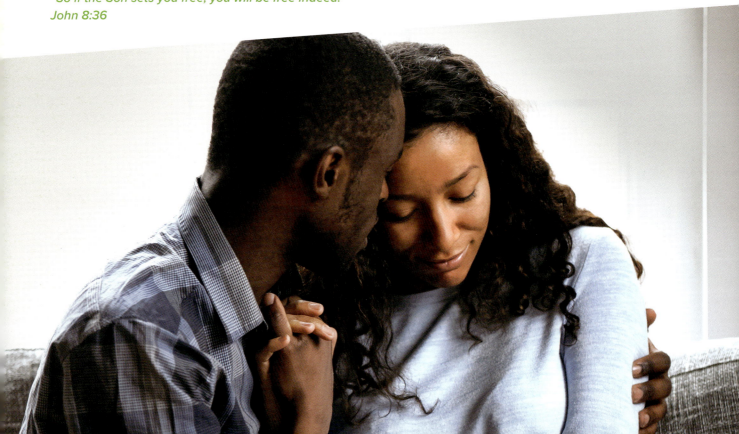

IN YOUR OWN WORDS

Read the following verse and then write out what it says to you.

"Therefore, having been justified by faith, we have peace with God through our Lord Jesus Christ."
Romans 5:1

....

....

....

....

....

....

....

....

....

....

Becky Pippert writes, "In much of the Western world, the biggest problem is not skepticism but sentimentalism. Convictions have been transformed into clichés. Christian truths are unknown because they are too well known."

Christians can make this rest from unresolved guilt sound formulaic. Yet the process really is as basic as A, B, C.

In the end, the only way to really know this peace is to experience it for yourself. And you can by admitting to God that you need His help, believing that Jesus, the Son of God, came to save you from your sins and by committing your life to follow Him forever.

ADMIT:

"For all have sinned and fall short of the glory of God." Romans 3:23

BELIEVE:

"God so loved the world that He gave His only begotten Son, that whoever believes in Him should not perish but have everlasting life."
John 3:16

COMMIT:

"If you confess with your mouth the Lord Jesus and believe in your heart that God has raised Him from the dead, you will be saved." Romans 10:9

REST FROM WORRY

In the Bible, God commands us not to worry. Worry always drains, disables and exhausts us. There is never a good side to worry. In fact, worry is the absence of trust.

You may know someone who is a "professional worrier." They worry about their money, car, children and cat. They worry about unlocked doors, the Middle East, the shoes they just bought at the mall, their allergies acting up and what the neighbors might be thinking. They even worry about how they're worrying too much. Besides the huge toll on their health, are they aware of the pain that they cause their God? If your young child said, "I'm just not sure you can take care of me and I worry all the time," — wouldn't that break your heart? Wouldn't you try with all your might to reassure them? In the same way, God whispers continually, "My child, please, trust Me."

"Be anxious for nothing, but in everything by prayer and supplication, with thanksgiving, let your requests be made known to God; and the peace of God, which surpasses all understanding, will guard your hearts and minds through Christ Jesus." Philippians 4:6, 7

Worries differ from valid concerns, but some people have a difficult time telling the two apart. Here's the principle difference between a worry and a valid concern: *can you do something about it?* If you can, then do it. If you can't, then pray about it and leave it in God's trustworthy hands.

"There is no fear in love; but perfect love casts out fear, because fear involves torment. But he who fears has not been made perfect in love." 1 John 4:18

Do we really, truly believe perfect love casts out *all* fear? Jesus, the Prince of Peace, places a hand on our shoulder and says softly, "Grace and peace to you." He heals us of our worrisome infirmity. Learning to count our blessings is the first step.

> There was once in China a woman who approached a wise man for advice. The woman was filled with anger and resentment. She asked the wise man, "Why has life been so cruel to me? Why must I suffer so? How can I go on living?"
>
> The wise man did not answer the woman's questions. Instead he told her, "Enter a house where no suffering has taken place, and ask them your questions."
>
> Three days later the woman returned. Her face now radiated a peaceful calm.
>
> "Tell me," said the wise man, "what did you find? And who answered your questions?"
>
> The woman said, "For three days I inquired from house to house throughout the city. Try as I might I could find no house without suffering. I heard so many stories of heartache, of great loss and terrible pain that I finally came to realize something. I have been most blessed in life."

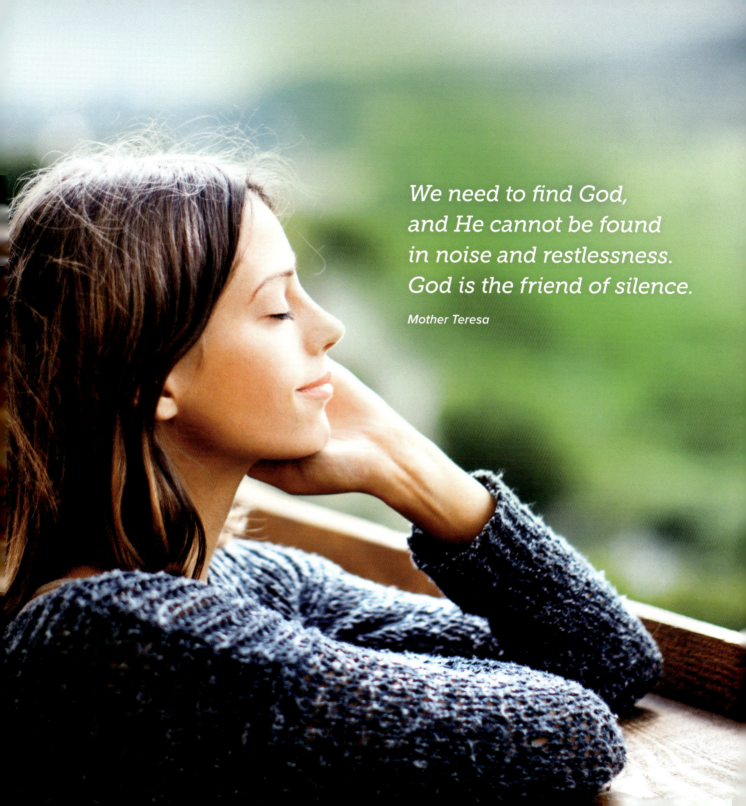

*We need to find God,
and He cannot be found
in noise and restlessness.
God is the friend of silence.*

Mother Teresa

CHECK IT OUT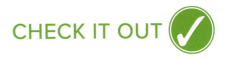

I FEEL MOST PEACEFUL WHEN I'M

- ☐ **CREATING SOMETHING OF BEAUTY.**
- ☐ **RELAXING WITH FRIENDS.**
- ☐ **TRULY BEING MYSELF.**
- ☐ **DOING WHAT I KNOW IS RIGHT.**
- ☐ **IN NATURE.**
- ☐ **HELPING SOMEONE.**
- ☐ **LISTENING TO MY MUSIC.**
- ☐ **TALKING WITH GOD.**
- ☐

STRESS REACTIONS

Harvard physiologist Dr. Walter Cannon performed a classic experiment studying a cat's vital functions when confronted by a dog. He found the following changes in the cat took place:

- Increased circulation
- More energy-rich sugar appeared in its blood
- Blood-clotting mechanisms accelerated
- Muscle functions increased
- Breathing quickened
- Senses became keener
- Unneeded digestive system shut down

These adaptive changes enhanced the cat's likelihood of survival. All of the cat's reactions were *involuntary*. The cat didn't make a conscious choice to speed up its circulation — it's just the way the cat was designed to react to the presence of a potential threat. All of the changes actually helped the cat achieve two possible reactions: fight back or run. This "fight or flight" response is present in all animals, even humans.

Whenever we encounter emergencies, our bodies respond much like the cat in Dr. Cannon's experiment. We don't arch our backs, expose our toenails and hiss, but all of the other involuntary responses happen inside with every emergency we perceive.

Now, what if the cat used these responses ten hours a day — for ten years? And what if the cat *never used* the responses for actually fighting or running? What would happen to that cat? Some people go through life racing and battling as if a monster dog were attacking them all the time. Can you imagine the toll it takes?

During the U.S. Civil War, a severe anxiety condition was documented called "soldier's heart." During World War I, soldiers termed it "shell shock." By World War II it was known as "battle fatigue." Vietnam War veterans were diagnosed with "post-traumatic stress disorder" (PTSD). We now know each of these illnesses was caused by a never-ending "fight or flight" environment.

But you're not in a war — or are you? Are you involved in never-ending battles with finances, job pressures and family problems? Then you're experiencing stress in a modern "civilized" war. Those prolonged stress responses often result in chronic suppression of the immune system.

Stress is now known to be a major contributor, either directly or indirectly, to coronary heart disease, cancer, strokes, lung ailments and accidental injuries — five of the leading causes of death in modern societies.

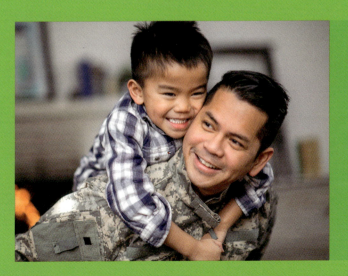

It is better to waste a minute of your life than to waste your life in a minute. Author Unknown

*"Rest in the Lord, and wait patiently for Him;
do not fret because of him who prospers in his way,
because of the man who brings wicked schemes to
pass. Cease from anger, and forsake wrath;
do not fret — it only causes harm. For evildoers
shall be cut off; but those who wait on the Lord,
they shall inherit the earth."* *Psalm 37:79*

God wants us to rest in Him. In other words, slow
down. Relax. Trust. Go forward in peace, by grace,
for love, with joy.

*"Cast all your anxieties upon Him,
for He cares about you."* *1 Peter 5:7*

No matter what our personal struggle is, God wants
to hear about it. God longs to guide us every step of
the way to healing and restoration.

REMEMBER THIS

**WRITE A BIBLE PROMISE FROM THIS REST
SECTION THAT YOU WOULD LIKE TO COMMIT
TO MEMORY TO HELP YOU THROUGH THE
CHALLENGES OF LIFE.**

....

....

....

....

....

....

*"'Fear not, for I am with you; be not dismayed, for I am
your God. I will strengthen you, yes, I will help you.'"*
Isaiah 41:10

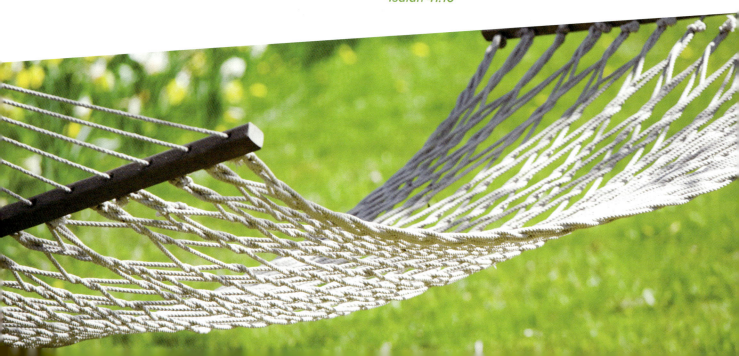

SABBATH REST

A young fighter pilot believed he didn't require an oxygen mask up to twenty thousand feet. He could function just fine without it, thank you. His superiors, decided to show him. They placed him in a low-oxygen chamber that simulated air at twenty thousand feet. After a few minutes, they asked him to write his full name, address, family's names, social security number and phone number on a pad of paper.

Upon exiting, the pilot grinned. He felt fine — no problem. Then he looked at what he had written and stared. The last three items were total gibberish — incomprehensible scrawling. He hadn't known his state at all.

Like the pilot, we function each week in rarefied, depleted air. Often we don't realize our true condition. The life-giving oxygen masks of prayer, the Bible and Sabbath enable us to legibly live God's love.

"Remember the Sabbath day, to keep it holy. Six days you shall labor and do all your work, but the seventh day is the Sabbath of the Lord your God. In it you shall do no work: you, nor your son, nor your daughter, nor your male servant, nor your female servant, nor your cattle, nor your stranger who is within your gates. For in six days the Lord made the heavens and the earth, the sea, and all that is in them, and rested the seventh day. Therefore the Lord blessed the Sabbath day and hallowed it." Exodus 20:8-11

> *They must realize that the Sabbath is the Lord's gift to you.* Exodus 16:29

Bombarded by amusements, we lose time for deepening, thoughtful reflection. In a famous passage about withdrawing to Walden Pond, Henry David Thoreau wrote, "I went to the woods because I wished to live deliberately, to front only the essential facts of life and see if I could not learn what it had to teach, and not, when I came to die, discover that I had not lived."

Of course, in the woods Thoreau didn't have to deal with a spouse, children, a demanding job and a million pressures in a culture based on expediency. With all our responsibilities, how can we leave and do what Thoreau did?

Sabbath is our "Walden Pond". Each week we can clear our minds, like rinsing a brush after painting, because we know the next job won't be as good if we don't clean our tools thoroughly. The Sabbath enables us to live deliberately and face the "essential facts of life." Sabbath brings us back to grace, delight and life.

Our society weighs our worth by how much and what we produce — quantity and quality. But on the Sabbath day God says, "Produce nothing. Now, hear this: I love you *just as much* today as on any workday. You are worth the world to Me just as you are because of who you are. My child, take a break from your striving."

Sabbath is an antidote to legalism, the belief that we somehow earn our way to God's love. One new Sabbath keeper reflects, "We started out our search with the desire for simplicity and an appreciation for rest. But the thing that really convinced me about Sabbath keeping was a friend who said, 'God didn't change any of the other commandments, so why would He have changed the fourth one?' The rationale behind that argument seems pretty airtight."

Call the Sabbath a delight. Isaiah 58:13

In his book *Velvet Elvis*, Rob Bell rhapsodizes about Sabbath:

> Sabbath is taking a day a week to remind myself that I did not make the world and that it will continue to exist without my efforts.

> Sabbath is a day when my work is done, even if it isn't.

> Sabbath is a day when my job is to enjoy. Period.

> Sabbath is a day when I am fully available to myself and to those I love most.

> Sabbath is a day when I remember that when God made the world, He saw that it was good.

> Sabbath is a day when I produce nothing.

> Sabbath is a day when I remind myself that I am not a machine.

> Sabbath is a day when at the end I say, "I didn't do anything today," and I don't add, "And I feel so guilty."

> Sabbath is a day when my phone is turned off, I don't check my e-mail and you can't get a hold of me.

> Jesus wants to heal our souls, wants to give us the Shalom of God. And so we have to stop. We have to slow down. We have to sit still and stare out the window and let the engine come to an idle. We have to listen to what our inner voice is saying.

"If you turn back your foot from the Sabbath, from doing your [business] on my holy day, and call the Sabbath a delight and the holy day of the Lord honorable; if you honor it, not going your own ways, or [pursuing your own business], or talking idly; then you shall take delight in the Lord, and I will make you ride upon the heights of the earth." Isaiah 58:13, 14

Have you ever shopped for a variety of different people? Think of it: *What could God have given everyone that would be just right?* God chose the perfect gift of time. Each week the Sabbath provides us with a sanctuary, a buried treasure in our sand-blown age.

As Abraham Heschel reports, the Sabbath is "a realm of time where the goal is not to have but to be, not to own but to give, not to control but to share, not to subdue but to be in accord. Life goes wrong when the control of space, the acquisition of the things of space, becomes our sole concern."

This rhythm of life originated back in Genesis in the Creation story. It is here that we discover God's design for us to rest on the seventh day of the week. The biblical Sabbath day of rest begins Friday evening at sundown and continues to Saturday at sundown. The Sabbath is a day for worship, reflection, prayer, recreation and mercy. It's a time to connect with the Creator and those around us.

"And He said to them, 'The Sabbath was made for man, and not man for the Sabbath. Therefore the Son of Man is also Lord of the Sabbath.'" Mark 2:27, 28

Sabbath is also the antidote to self-addiction. As we make time for God, family and close friends, we reconnect with eternal matters. Resting from ourselves, we become our true selves again.

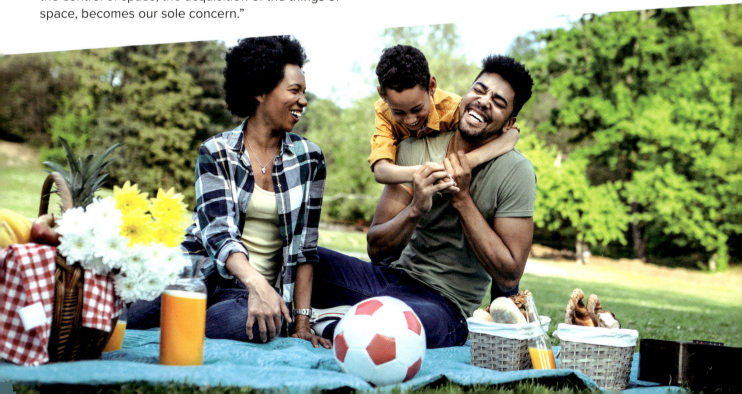

Of course we still battle against the demands placed upon as by the hands of the clock. The "world" will always break into the Sabbath rhythm if we allow it. Eugene Peterson writes,

> The "world" is sometimes our friends, sometimes our families, sometimes our employers — they want us to work for them, not waste time with God, not be our original selves. If the world can get rid of Sabbath, it has us to itself. What it does with us when it gets us is not very attractive: after a few years of Sabbath breaking we are passive consumers of expensive trash, and anxious hurriers after fantasy pleasures. We lose our God and our dignity at about the same time.

We can't seem to stand the thought of letting the newspaper go unread or another bargain slide by — we see added things to do, find more ways to "get ahead." Tilden Edwards claims "stopping work tests our trust: will the world and I fall apart if I stop making things happen for a while?" *In My Fair Lady*, Eliza Doolittle accents an apt response: "Without your twirling it the earth still spins, without your pulling it the tide rolls in, without your pushing them the clouds roll by."

The wonder is that even Christians miss this Sabbath rest. They don't realize the gift Jesus intends when He promises, "Come to me, all who labor and are heavy laden, and I will give you rest."

God in effect assures us every Sabbath, "You are a human being, not a human doing or a human done. You are priceless because I have paid infinity for you. You are My child. I will never leave or forget you. Your name is graven on the palms of My hands." (See Isaiah 49:15, 16.)

JESUS AND SABBATH

"So He came to Nazareth, where He had been brought up. And as His custom was, He went into the synagogue on the Sabbath day, and stood up to read." Luke 4:16

Though Jesus often entered into controversy with religious leaders over the Sabbath, the battles were never over *whether* the day should be kept, or even which day should be kept. Instead the battle was always and only over *how* it was to be kept. The Sabbath had become a burden, and Jesus wanted people to see that the Sabbath was made for their benefit, to give them rest and peace in Him, both physically and spiritually.

"'For the Son of Man is Lord even of the Sabbath.' Now when [Jesus] had departed from there, He went into their synagogue. And behold, there was a man who had a withered hand. And they asked Him, saying, 'Is it lawful to heal on the Sabbath? — that they might accuse Him.

Then He said to them, 'What man is there among you who has one sheep, and if it falls into a pit on the Sabbath, will not lay hold of it and lift it out? 'Of how much more value then is a man than a sheep? Therefore it is lawful to do good on the Sabbath.' Then He said to the man, 'Stretch out your hand.' And he stretched it out, and it was restored as whole." Matthew 12:8-13

Sabbath is a marvelous day for mercy.

IN YOUR OWN WORDS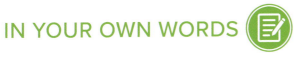

WRITE SOME THOUGHTS ABOUT HOW YOU CAN KEEP THE SABBATH AND THE BENEFITS THIS WILL BRING TO YOU.

....

....

....

....

....

....

....

....

....

SOS — SAVE OUR SLEEP

According to the National Sleep Foundation, more than 100 million people in the United States suffer from sleep deprivation. More than 40 percent of these sleep each night less than six hours. How can we break the restless cycle?

Research has found that sleep during the hours before midnight is more beneficial than sleep taken after midnight.

Research also demonstrates that going to bed earlier to get enough sleep helps our immune systems and brains to function optimally and to make healthy choices. Sleep improves creativity; memory; blood pressure and inflammation; athletic performance; longevity; desired weight loss, driving (fewer accidents); stress levels; and overall well-being.

What other activity gives us such amazing health benefits? Feeling uncreative, forgetful, stressed, exhausted or depressed? Try *sleep*.

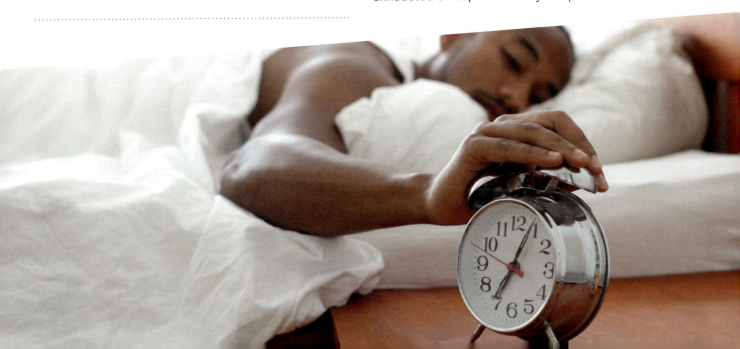

TIPS FOR BETTER SLEEP

1. **Use "progressive muscle relaxation."** Tense a group of muscles as you deeply breathe in through your nose, and relax them as you slowly breathe out through your mouth. Start with your hands, and work your way down your body — arms, shoulders, neck, jaw, eyes, abdomen, back, legs and feet. Ensure before moving on that all the other muscle groups are continuing to be relaxed.

2. **Get adequate sunlight, fresh air and physical activity during the day.** Research shows your sleep at night may suffer if your body doesn't receive all of these.

3. **Limit daytime naps to 20 minutes.** "Power naps" have been shown to possess many benefits, including enhancing alertness, memory, calmness and performance. Longer naps, however, can make sleeping at night difficult.

4. **Avoid caffeine, tobacco and other stimulants.** Also, because digestion keeps the body active, don't eat anything within three hours of going to sleep.

5. **Establish regular sleep patterns.** Try going to bed at the same time each night and getting up the same time each morning. Staying up late or sleeping in more than 30 minutes on the weekend disrupts your weekly sleep pattern. In addition, use the bed only for sleep and intimacy. Doing other activities — such as paying bills and reading — "teaches" the body to remain awake when in bed.

6. **Relax during the last hour at night.** Keep conflict, anxiety and stress outside your bedroom. (No television, video games or aggravating Internet blogs). Many find it especially restful to take a hot bath.

7. **Keep your room dark, quiet, cool and comfortable.** Experiencing an optimal atmosphere, including a mattress and pillow that are right for you, can make all the difference in getting a good night's sleep.

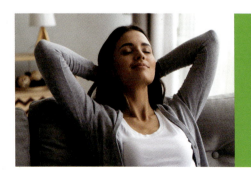

Sometimes the most urgent and vital thing you can possibly do is take a complete rest. Ashleigh Brilliant

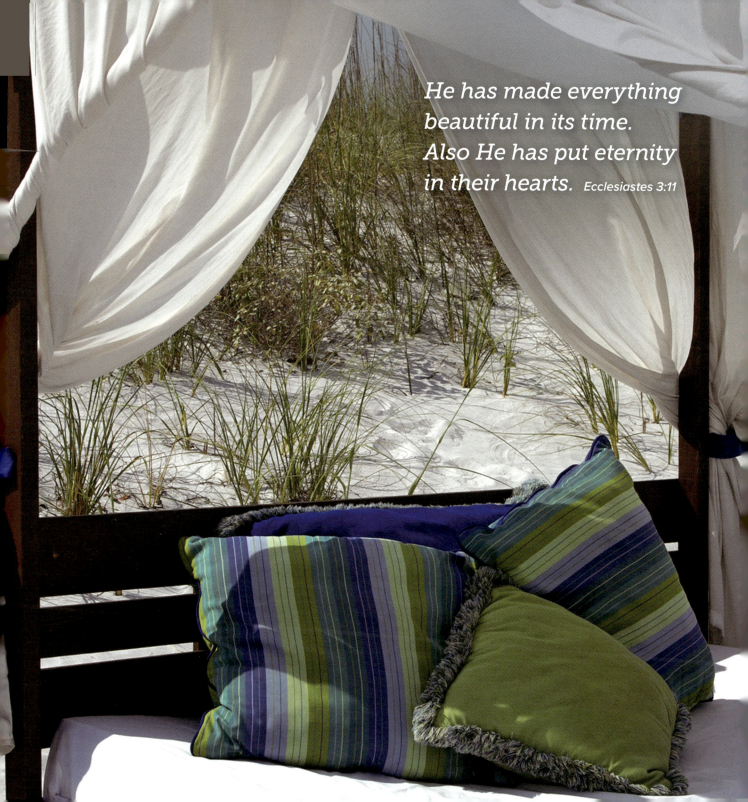

He has made everything beautiful in its time. Also He has put eternity in their hearts. *Ecclesiastes 3:11*

MORNING HAS BROKEN

Finally, one healthy choice is to commit our lives to God at the beginning of the day. When we stay up late we are less likely to be able to (or want to) get up with enough time to connect with God.

"And Abraham went early in the morning to the place where he had stood before the Lord." *Genesis 19:27*

"But I will sing of Your power; yes, I will sing aloud of Your mercy in the morning; for You have been my defense and refuge in the day of my trouble."
Psalm 59:16

"Now in the morning, having risen a long while before daylight, He went out and departed to a solitary place; and there He prayed." *Mark 1:35*

Here we see Abraham, David and Jesus getting up early and connecting with God. Won't you consider making the same powerfully positive choice? Recall the original days of Genesis 1: "So the evening and the morning were the fourth day" (verse 19). Note that the day begins at sundown. What if you began your days "the night before"? Wouldn't you be more organized, more prepared, more *rested*?

If you are not currently getting up early, start small by getting up 15 minutes earlier and have a short devotional time. This will energize and empower your day. God will bless you in your efforts to connect with Him and improve your life.

"My voice You shall hear in the morning, O Lord; in the morning I will direct it to You, and I will look up."
Psalm 5:3

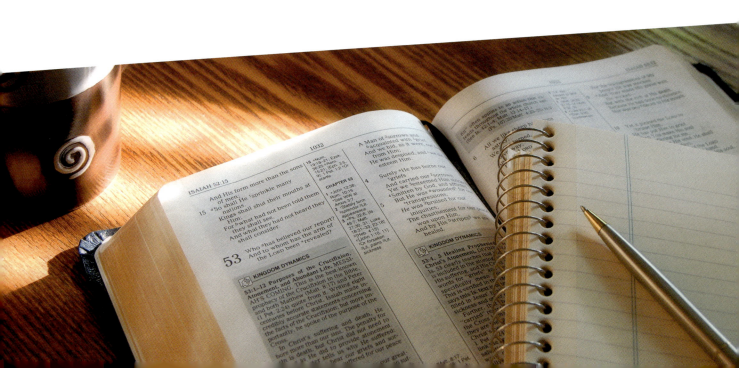

WHERE DO YOU FIND THE TIME?

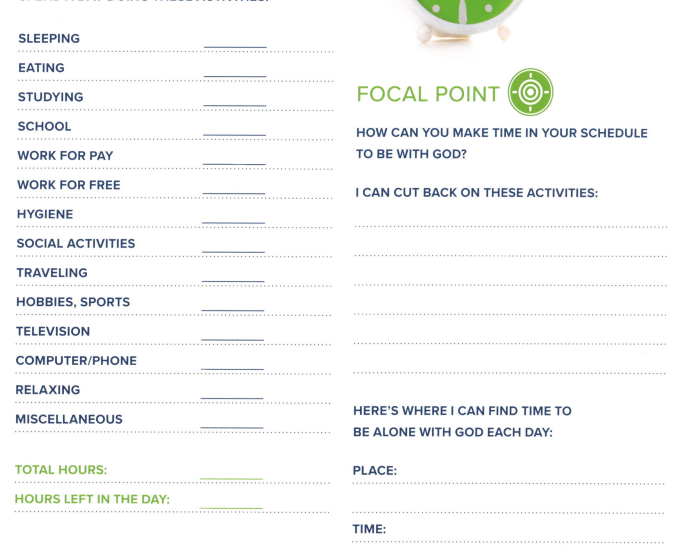

WRITE DOWN THE NUMBER OF HOURS YOU
SPEND A DAY DOING THESE ACTIVITIES:

SLEEPING _____

EATING _____

STUDYING _____

SCHOOL _____

WORK FOR PAY _____

WORK FOR FREE _____

HYGIENE _____

SOCIAL ACTIVITIES _____

TRAVELING _____

HOBBIES, SPORTS _____

TELEVISION _____

COMPUTER/PHONE _____

RELAXING _____

MISCELLANEOUS _____

TOTAL HOURS: _____

HOURS LEFT IN THE DAY: _____

FOCAL POINT

HOW CAN YOU MAKE TIME IN YOUR SCHEDULE
TO BE WITH GOD?

I CAN CUT BACK ON THESE ACTIVITIES:

....

....

....

....

....

HERE'S WHERE I CAN FIND TIME TO
BE ALONE WITH GOD EACH DAY:

PLACE:
....

TIME:
....

LIFE APPLICATION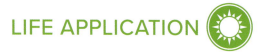

Take a moment to reflect on this CREATION Life study on rest.

WHAT PRINCIPLES HAVE YOU LEARNED THAT YOU WANT TO APPLY IN YOUR LIFE?

....

....

....

....

NOW, CREATE A PERSONAL GOAL FOR REST.

....

....

....

....

Examples of a goals for rest:

My goal is to be a peacemaker this week by listening to others, choosing a soft answer, staying reasonable and treating everyone with kindness.

My goal is to recite a Bible text and/or sing a hymn, and wait patiently for God each time I'm tempted to worry this week.

My goal is to enjoy God's rest every Sabbath, beginning this week.

My goal is to get 7-8 hours of solid sleep each night.

My goal is to get up 15 minutes earlier every day this week to spend time in prayer and Bible study with God.

SMALL GROUP DISCUSSION QUESTIONS

1. **WHAT BIBLE TEXT ON REST IMPACTED YOU MOST IN THIS SECTION?**

....

....

2. **HOW DO YOU THINK "SHALOM RIPPLES" CAN CHANGE YOUR WORLD AND YOUR FAMILY?**

....

....

3. SHARE A BIBLE PROMISE YOU WANT TO REMEMBER.

....

....

4. DO YOU KNOW A "PROFESSIONAL WORRIER?" WHAT HELPS YOU
   TO STOP WORRYING? SHARE SPECIFIC TECHNIQUES WITH THE GROUP.

....

....

5. EUGENE PETERSON WRITES, "IF THE WORLD CAN GET RID OF SABBATH, IT HAS US TO ITSELF."
   WHAT DOES THIS THOUGHT MEAN TO YOU? HOW COULD YOU CELEBRATE SABBATH?

....

....

6. WHAT REST PRINCIPLE IN YOUR LIFE APPLICATION STOOD OUT FOR YOU?

....

....

7. SHARE ONE REST GOAL WITH THE GROUP. ARE YOU FEELING CONFIDENT ABOUT REACHING YOUR
   GOAL? HOW CAN WE HELP ONE ANOTHER TO REACH OUR GOALS?

....

....

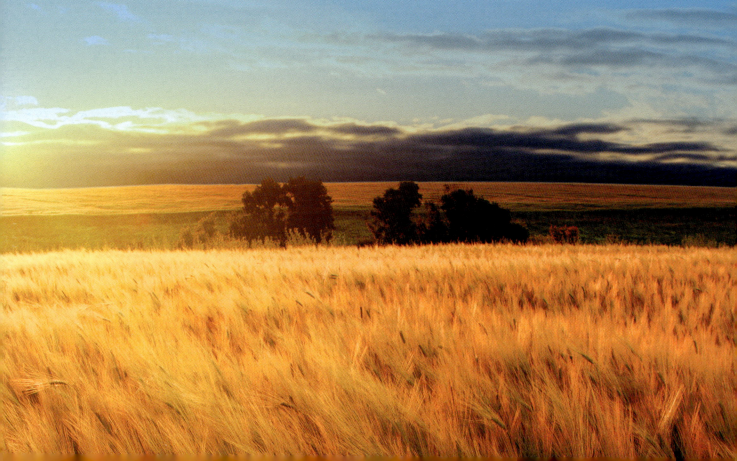

For by Him all things were created that are in heaven and that are on earth, visible and invisible... All things were created through Him and for Him. **Colossians 1:16**

ENVIRONMENT

When you think of "environment," what images come to mind? Do you immediately picture our blue-green planet rotating on its axis? Do you visualize the many ecosystems our world has to offer — rainforests, coral reefs and deserts? Do your thoughts fly to the scarcity of our natural resources and the importance of conservation?

There's no doubt that environment exerts a powerful impact on our bodies and minds. Whether soaring eagles above towering redwoods or tadpoles changing into croaking bullfrogs, nature is majestic and miraculous. And yet, as founder of the modern environmental movement Rachel Carson describes, too often we take it all for granted.

> My companion and I were alone with the stars: the misty river of the Milky Way flowing across the sky, the patterns of the constellations standing out bright and clear, a blazing planet low on the horizon. It occurred to me that if this were a sight that could be seen only once in a century, this little headland would be thronged with spectators. But it can be seen many scores of nights in any year, and so the lights burned in the cottages and the inhabitants probably gave not a thought to the beauty overhead; and because they could see it almost any night, perhaps they never will.

Often we don't see what is right in front of us. We fix our gaze on tiny screens, content to live a virtual life while the real beauty God created goes ignored and overlooked. Of course, our environment can also be trash-strewn streets and concrete buildings with jarring noises. Many of us have exchanged a natural environment for an oppressive, urban one. But are we really better off? Are we experiencing abundant life in cubicles and shopping malls? How can we enjoy an environment where love, freedom, joy and beauty flourish?

Where I Am (*Place a mark on the line to show what you're feeling right now.*)

My environment tends
to depress me.

My environment fills me with
wonder and delight.

IN THE BEGINNING...

From the start, our environment was *good*. We were created for goodness sake from the hand of our good Creator.

The world God created provided every living thing with optimal surroundings. Beauty filled even the smallest, simplest acts of nature.

In *Pilgrim at Tinker Creek,* Annie Dillard relates such an act. At first glance, it appears to be another mundane occurrence, but something about the experience resonates with wonder.

About five years ago I saw a mockingbird make a straight vertical descent from the roof gutter of a four-story building. It was an act as careless and spontaneous as the curl of a stem or the kindling of a star. The mockingbird took a single step into the air and dropped. His wings were still folded against his sides as though he were singing from a limb and not falling, accelerating thirty-two feet per second through empty air. Just a breath before he would have been dashed to the ground, he unfurled his wings with exact, deliberate care, revealing the broad bars of white, spread his elegant, white-banded tail and so floated onto the grass.

She concludes, "Beauty and grace are performed whether or not we will or sense them. The least we can do is try to be there."

Adam and Eve were there, eyewitnesses to God's beauty and grace revealed everyday in their environment. God wants us to be there too. By experiencing the wonders of creation we can reconnect to our Creator and live a life permeated with marvels.

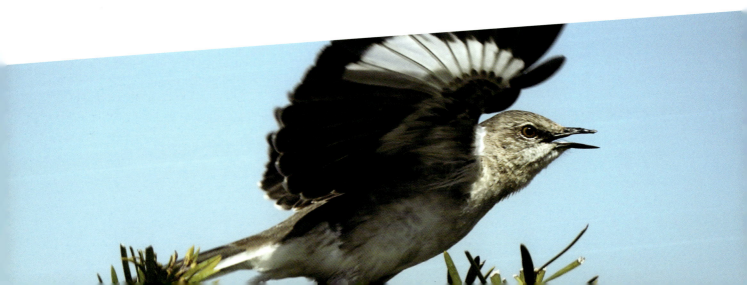

In her book *Packing for Mars: The Curious Science of Life in the Void* (2010), Mary Roach examines the effects of being disconnected from the earth.

> I once met a man who told me that after landing in Christchurch, New Zealand, after a winter at the South Pole research station, he and his companions spent a couple days just wandering around staring in awe at flowers and trees. At one point, one of them spotted a woman pushing a stroller. *"A baby!"* he shouted, and they all rushed across the street to see. The woman turned the stroller and ran.

After months surrounded by frozen barrenness, the men were amazed at the simple sights of nature. Roach goes on to explain how an unnatural environment creates in all of us a longing to return to nature.

> Nothing tops space as a barren, unnatural environment. Astronauts who had no prior interest in gardening spend hours tending experimental greenhouses. "They are our love," said cosmonaut Vladislav Volkov of the tiny flax plants with which they shared the confines of Salyut 1, the first Soviet space station.

> Humans don't belong in space…. Weightlessness is an exhilarating novelty, but floaters soon begin to dream of walking. Earlier [Alexandr] Laveikin told us, "Only in space do you understand what incredible happiness it is just to walk. To walk on Earth."

IN YOUR OWN WORDS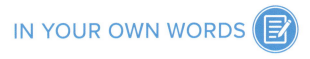

WHAT IN NATURE DO YOU TEND TO TAKE FOR GRANTED?

....
....
....
....
....
....

"Then the Lord God took the man and put him in the Garden of Eden to tend and keep it." Genesis 2:15

God gave the earth for us to enjoy and be blessed by it, and He also gave us the environment to use as a resource. Animals, plants and minerals provide us with helpful materials for growth and prosperity. However, God never intended for us to abuse these resources. The best modern description of our job assignment is *caretaker* — a person who is in charge of the maintenance of an area.

> God wants us to be caretakers of the environment that surrounds us. He designed it to sustain us: air to breathe, sunshine to warm and heal us and food and water to eat and drink. God yearns for us to treasure this planet we call home.

DETERIORATING ENVIRONMENT

"For the creation was subjected to futility, not of its own will but by the will of him who subjected it in hope; because the creation itself also will be set free from its bondage to decay and obtain the glorious liberty of the children of God. We know that the whole creation has been groaning in travail together until now."
Romans 8:20-22

Humankind's continual use of the earth has also changed it. Every day we hear about deforestation, climate change, habitat encroachment and other environmental issues. Through constant use and misuse, our environment has deteriorated over millennia.

In his 2009 book *Threshold*, Thom Hartmann paints a grim picture facing our planet, including the disturbing fact that "today more than three billion of the world's nearly seven billion people don't have reliable access to safe water, sanitation or food supplies." From the chapter entitled "The Environment," he writes:

> With a human population pushing past seven billion and the number of humans who eat a meat/fish rich diet (versus mostly a plant-rich diet) moving from under a billion to more than three billion (each consuming between ten and thirty times the basic plant protein necessary to feed the livestock)... the capacity of the planet to carry this huge burden is rapidly becoming exhausted.

FOCAL POINT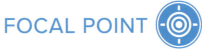

WHAT DO YOU THINK IS OUR PLANET'S MOST PRESSING ENVIRONMENTAL PROBLEM?

....

....

....

....

....

....

....

"'The nations raged, but thy wrath came, and the time for the dead to be judged, for rewarding thy servants, the prophets and saints, and those who fear thy name, both small and great, and for destroying the destroyers of the earth.'" Revelation 11:18

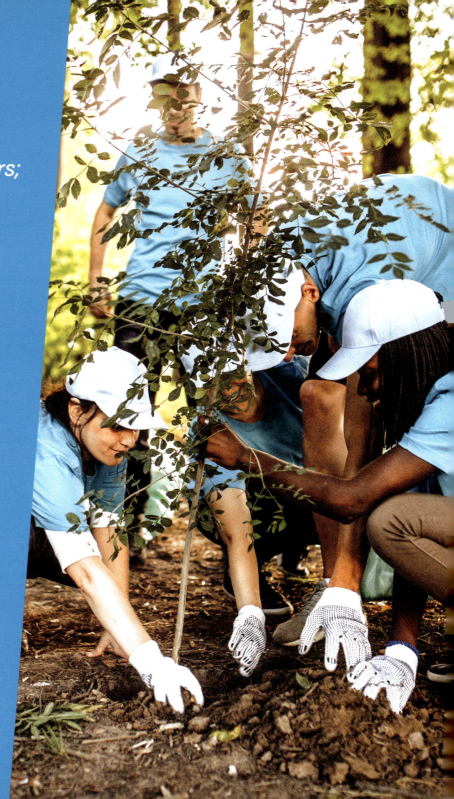

We do not inherit the earth from our ancestors; we borrow it from our children. **Chief Seattle**

"But now ask the beasts, and they will teach you; and the birds of the air, and they will tell you; or speak to the earth, and it will teach you; and the fish of the sea will explain to you. Who among all these does not know that the hand of the Lord has done this?" Job 12:7-9

God intends for us to learn from the natural world. After all, nature has been called God's second book, and it has much to teach us.

The Bible assures us that creation reveals the work of God.

"Since the creation of the world His invisible attributes are clearly seen, being understood by the things that are made." Romans 1:20

This means when we look at nature, we glimpse His majestic power and intricate artistry. God has put them on display for all people to witness everyday.

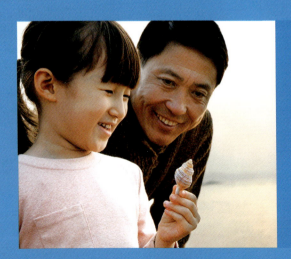

The heavens declare the glory of God; and the firmament shows His handiwork.

Psalm 19:1

But what about when nature frightens us? When earthquakes, tsunamis, tornados, floods and hurricanes hit, how do we relate to God? Is God behind those natural horrors as well?

When disaster strikes, many find it difficult to reconcile the pictures of destruction with the idea of a loving, caring God. Some even view these events as God's judgment upon the evil of the world. Religious leaders from across the spectrum use these tragedies as opportunities to speculate wildly. The phrases "divine judgment" and "retribution" are tossed about, sparking controversy and outrage.

We tend to think that life here should be fair because God is fair. But God is not life here. God is behind life. He is the Author of life, the Hope of life and the End of life. A painter, while "seen" in her painting, is not the painting itself. She will especially not be seen in the work when her enemies have the ability to spoil it.

Life here is like the backside of a tapestry, its threads all jumbled with indistinct, muted colors and clashing patterns. We can sort of make out the picture. But it's not until we get on the front side of the tapestry, the other side of life here, that we experience the full design, the reason for every knotted red, gray, black and white thread. Only then can we truly see what the Master Artist has created.

No matter what we may face in this life, we can "know that all things work together for good to those who love God" (Romans 8:28). In all circumstances, we can know that nothing — neither disease, drought, devil or death — will be able to separate us from the love of God.

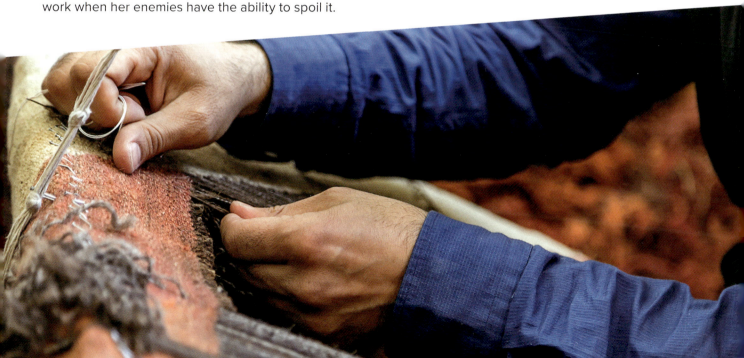

IN YOUR OWN WORDS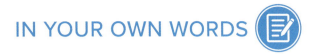

WHAT SHOULD WE KEEP IN MIND
WHEN LIFE IS NOT FAIR?

....

....

....

....

....

....

....

....

....

Frank S. Mead tells a parable to illustrate how nature reveals the trustworthiness of God.

> Nasr-ed-Din Hodja, in the heat of the day, sat under a walnut tree looking at his pumpkin vines. He said to himself, "How foolish God is! Here He puts a great heavy pumpkin on a tiny vine without strength to do anything but lie on the ground. And He puts a tiny walnut on tree whose branches could hold the weight of a man. If I were God, I could do a better job than that!"

> Just then a breeze dislocated a walnut in the tree, and it fell on the head of skeptical Nasr-ed-Din Hodja, who rubbed his head a sadder and wiser man. "Suppose," he mused, "there had been a pumpkin up there instead of a walnut. Never again will I try to plan the world for God, but I shall thank God that He has done so well."

MAKING SENSE OF OUR ENVIRONMENT

As human beings we're incredibly complex, with more than a trillion cellular interactions in our bodies every second. One of the best ways to maintain a good focus is to fill our senses with good stimuli. Whatever we see, hear, smell, touch and taste in our environment will be what we naturally perceive and think about.

How does the Bible encourage us to fill our senses?

SIGHT

"My child, give me your heart,
and let your eyes observe my ways."
Proverbs 23:26

Concentrate not on your trials and discouragements, but rather on Jesus and His strength. Consider this example from Scripture.

"Immediately Jesus made His disciples get into the boat and go before Him to the other side, while He sent the multitudes away. And when He had sent the multitudes away, He went up on the mountain by Himself to pray. Now when evening came, He was alone there. But the boat was now in the middle of the sea, tossed by the waves, for the wind was contrary. Now in the fourth watch of the night Jesus went to them, walking on the sea. And when the disciples saw Him walking on the sea, they were troubled, saying, 'It is a ghost!' And they cried out for fear. But immediately Jesus spoke to them, saying, 'Be of good cheer! It is I; do not be afraid.' And Peter answered Him and said, 'Lord, if it is You, command me to come to You on the water.'

So He said, 'Come.' And when Peter had come down out of the boat, he walked on the water to go to Jesus. But when he saw that the wind was boisterous, he was afraid; and beginning to sink he cried out, saying, 'Lord, save me!' And immediately Jesus stretched out His hand and caught him, and said to him, 'O you of little faith, why did you doubt?' And when they got into the boat, the wind ceased. Then those who were in the boat came and worshiped Him, saying, 'Truly You are the Son of God.'" Matthew 14:22-33

As long as he kept his sight on Jesus, Peter walked on the water. But as soon as he took his eyes off Jesus and saw the waves crashing around him, he began sinking. When we turn our eyes on Jesus instead of our difficulties, He will give us strength.

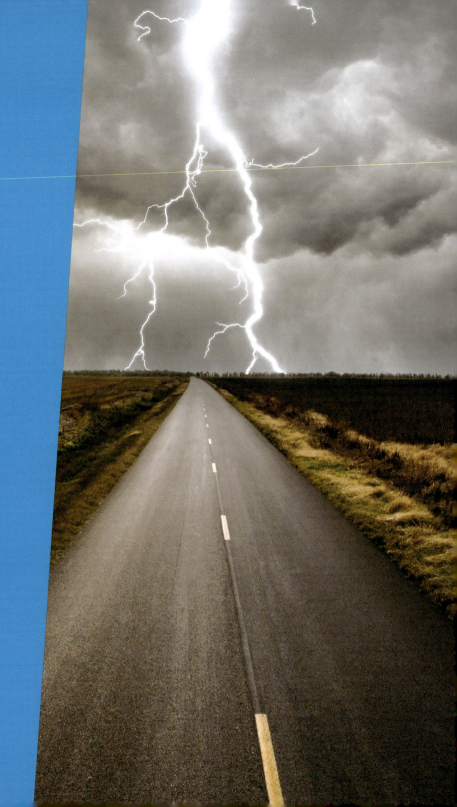

My Prayer: Jesus, Master and Friend, help me to focus on You rather than on the failures and struggles I experience in my environment. Give me the strength I need to endure the storms of life.

SMELL

The fig tree puts forth her green figs, and the vines with the tender grapes give a good smell. Rise up, my love, my fair one, and come away!"
Song of Solomon 2:13

"His branches shall spread; His beauty shall be like an olive tree, and his fragrance like Lebanon."
Hosea 14:6

Did you know the sense of smell is the closest sensory link to emotions and memories? Consider using aromatherapy to encourage your own relaxation and positive attitude.

Amazingly, the air inside our homes is an average of 2-5 times more polluted than the outside, and most Americans spend 90 percent of their time indoors. Indoor air pollution is caused by cleaning products, insecticides, personal care products and garbage. Of course we can use non-toxic products and scented candles, but the best approach is to open windows and doors, or even better, get outside in the fresh air.

HEARING

"He who covers a transgression seeks love, but he who repeats a matter separates friends."
Proverbs 17:9

"Let everyone be quick to listen, slow to speak, slow to anger." *James 1:19*

What we hear profoundly affects our stress level and attitude. Noise pollution — as well as unkind or harsh words — can produce negative effects while words of love, music, singing and sounds of nature can create positive results. Take a personal sound inventory and evaluate how you can minimize noise pollution in your life.

TOUCH

"And behold, a leper came and worshiped Him, saying, 'Lord, if You are willing, You can make me clean.' Then Jesus put out His hand and touched him, saying, 'I am willing; be cleansed.' Immediately his leprosy was cleansed." Matthew 8:2, 3

Touch helps infants to develop, and it also helps children and adults to possess a greater sense of calm. Additionally, those who regularly hug or are hugged appear to have better health.

Jesus gave us an example of touch. In many of His miracles He insisted on touching people, and they were made whole. Jesus wanted to heal people in every way — spiritually, socially, physically and emotionally.

Jesus stretched out His hand and caught him.

Matthew 14:31

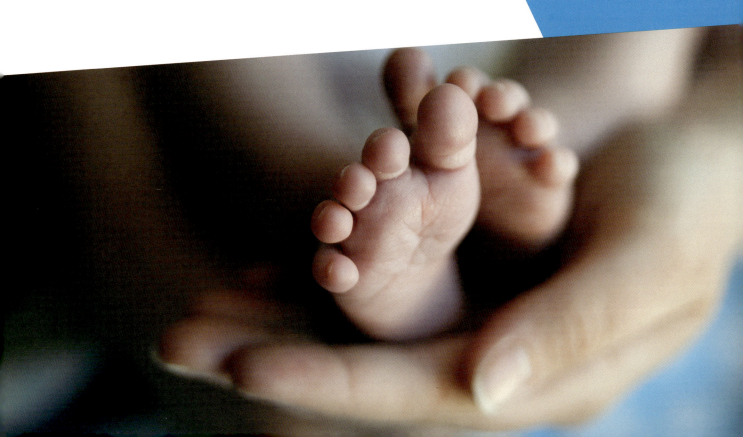

"He touched her hand, and the fever left her."
Matthew 8:15

"All those who had any that were sick were brought to Him; and He laid His hands on every one of them and healed them."   *Luke 4:40*

"The whole multitude sought to touch Him, for power went out from Him and healed them all."   *Luke 6:19*

"Then He came and touched the open coffin."
Luke 7:14

"He took her by the hand and said, 'My child, get up!'"
Luke 8:54

"Then He touched their eyes."   *Matthew 9:29*

"He... put His fingers in his ears, and He spat and touched his tongue."
Mark 7:33

"He took the blind man by the hand and led him out of the town."   *Mark 8:23*

"Jesus came and touched them. 'Get up,' he said. 'Don't be afraid.'"   *Matthew 17:7*

"But Jesus took him by the hand and lifted him up."
Mark 9:27

"He spit on the ground, made some mud with the saliva, and put it on the man's eyes."   *John 9:6*

"And He laid His hands on her, and immediately she was made straight, and glorified God."
Luke 13:13

"So taking hold of the man, He healed him."   *Luke 14:4*

"They also brought infants to Him that He might touch them."   *Luke 18:15*

"He poured water into a basin and began to wash the disciples' feet, and to wipe them with the towel."
John 13:5

"But Jesus answered and said, 'Permit even this.' And He touched his ear and healed him."   *Luke 22:51*

IN YOUR OWN WORDS

WHAT DO YOU LEARN ABOUT GOD FROM THESE VERSES ON TOUCH?

....

....

....

....

....

....

....

....

....

TASTE

"Can flavorless food be eaten without salt?
Or is there any taste in the white of an egg?"
Job 6:6

"My son, eat honey because it is good,
and the honeycomb which is sweet to your taste."
Proverbs 24:13

Eating is meant to be a pleasure. Take time to enjoy your food, whether it is savory, sweet, tart, warm, hot, cold, fresh, raw, baked or broiled. Savor every bite. Our food is our fuel, meant to energize us with vitality and health.

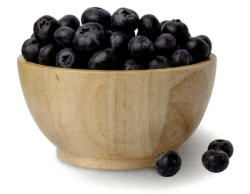

LIFE APPLICATION

Humans crave being around nature. Studies have found that the presence of windows, plants and natural sunlight creates a profound effect of productivity, healing, longevity and attitude. Many schools, hospitals, offices and even jail cells have used this to great effect. Urban neighborhoods also benefit from providing access to nature — parks, trees, plants, grass and water generate a calming effect that leads to fewer reports of violence and aggression, and strengthens community spirit.

So how can you change your environment for the better? How will you begin to integrate the beauty of nature into your life? Start by living with an attitude of gratitude. The next time you see a stunning sunset, hear a baby's giggle, taste a succulent salad, hug a friend or smell freshly baked bread, remember to say, *"Thank You, God."*

WHAT LIFE APPLICATIONS COME TO MIND FOR ENJOYING NATURE WITH YOUR SENSES MORE EACH DAY?

....

....

....

....

....

....

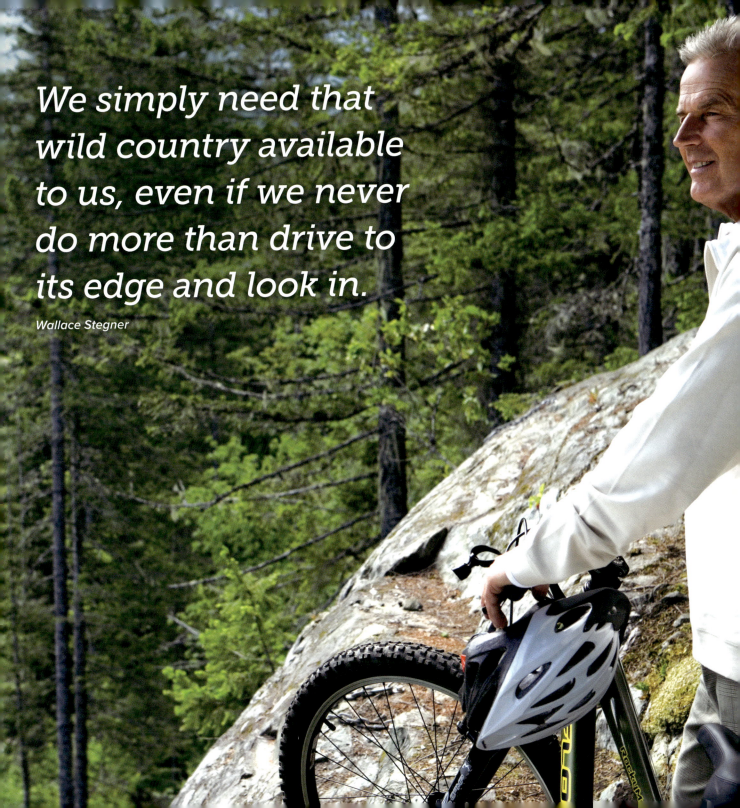

We simply need that wild country available to us, even if we never do more than drive to its edge and look in.

Wallace Stegner

NATURAL HEALTH ENHANCERS

SUNSHINE

"Truly the light is sweet, and a pleasant thing it is for the eyes to behold the sun."   Ecclesiastes 11:7

Truly, sunshine promotes happiness. Research has discovered sunshine increases serotonin, known as the "happy hormone." Furthermore, an imbalance of serotonin levels may lead to depression. This is why it's so important to spend some time outside in sunshine.

While we should take care not to become overexposed to ultraviolet rays, a review study came to this astounding conclusion: Although frequent regular exposure causes 2,000 U.S. cancer fatalities per year, sunlight also acts to prevent another annual 138,000 cancer deaths in the U.S.[1]

How often do you get out in the sunshine during any given week? Take precautions for overexposure and have fun in the sun.

FRESH AIR

"The Spirit of God has made me, and the breath of the Almighty gives me life."   Job 33:4

Fresh air is "negatively ionized," which is actually a good thing. Its benefits include improved function in the lung's protective cilia, decreased anxiety, improved learning and decreased survival of bacteria in the air. Some even use "negative air ionization therapy" to treat "seasonal affective disorder" (SAD).

However, often the air inside our homes is re-circulated. The more we breathe it the more we are losing the benefits God intended for us to enjoy with each breath. Try opening your windows and regularly getting outdoors to gain the maximum health benefits of fresh air.

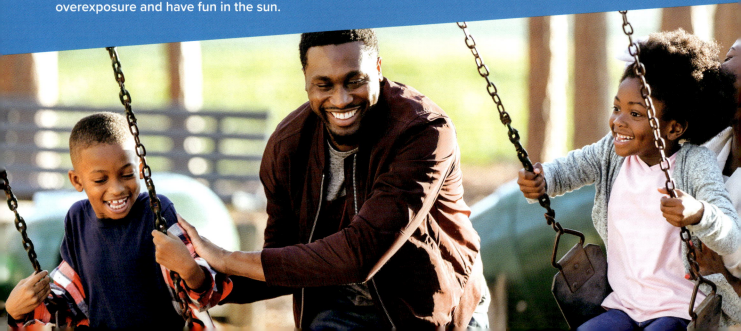

EARTH MADE NEW

"Now I saw a new heaven and a new earth, for the first heaven and the first earth had passed away. Also there was no more sea. Then I, John, saw the holy city, New Jerusalem, coming down out of heaven from God, prepared as a bride adorned for her husband.

And I heard a loud voice from heaven saying, 'Behold, the tabernacle of God is with men, and He will dwell with them, and they shall be His people. God Himself will be with them and be their God. And God will wipe away every tear from their eyes; there shall be no more death, nor sorrow, nor crying. There shall be no more pain, for the former things have passed away.'

Then He who sat on the throne said, 'Behold, I make all things new.'"   Revelation 21:1-5

Blaming the complexity of our lives on our environment, we may dream of getting away — perhaps to a remote island to relish the simple life. But, of course, the problem is not entirely our environment. The problem is in our anxious, disjointed lives. Because of sin, we are torn and aching. Life doesn't work for us regardless of what good things we choose to surround ourselves. We need a Savior.

The glorious good news is that eternal life — intimate friendship with God — is ours through Jesus. And eternal life begins here. Now.

"I write this to you who believe in the name of the Son of God, that you may know that you have eternal life." 1 John 5:13

Jesus provides us with hope for living. This hope becomes the melody of our song, one we sing whenever we feel lost or alone. At the end of life, the hopeful promise of being reunited with loved ones buoys us in the dark canyons of death's towering swells. Walter Lowen remembers,

> Let me tell you what the doctor who attended my wife did for me as I stood dazed and lost at the foot of her bed, knowing not only that the 37 years we had had together were over, but feeling also that all meaning had gone from life forever. He took my arm and held it for a moment. And then he said in a matter-of-fact voice: "You'll see her again."

That was all.

But it was all I needed to hear.

What is honored in a country will be cultivated there.

Plato

A REAL WORLD

We are not destined to recline on cumulous couches, strumming harps and eating angel food cake. Our home will be this earth made new. A place where we not only experience the beauty of nature as God intended it, but where we also cultivate and care for this home forever. This is why it is so important for us to take care of our home now. When we understand this, we know why environmentalism should be especially important to Christians.

The new earth will be second nature to us. As caretakers for the creation again, will we trash our home, brazenly wasting and poisoning resources? If not, then we must not trash this earth either. Our eternal home is beneath our feet.

In the afterlife, every good sensation will be intensified. Without the deadening shroud of sin, we will feel a thousand times stronger, see a thousand times deeper, communicate a thousand times clearer, hear a thousand times better and think a thousand times purer.

Think about what it means to be new earth people now. Are we choosing to invest in others? Are we enjoying the natural, creative and authentic? What will it be like to enter the land of beginning again? No wheelchair-accessible buildings, no cemetery plots, no barred windows, no groaning creation. We will truly return to Eden.

When Jesus died on the cross, He said, "It is finished!" Justice and mercy were fully demonstrated, Satan's charges were refuted and humanity was set free. But in the new earth the presence of sin — separation from God — is completely finished. Jesus frames this time in the sweetest words ever spoken to human ears:

"'Well done, good and faithful servant; you have been faithful over a few things, I will make you ruler over many things. Enter into the joy of your Lord."
Matthew 25:21

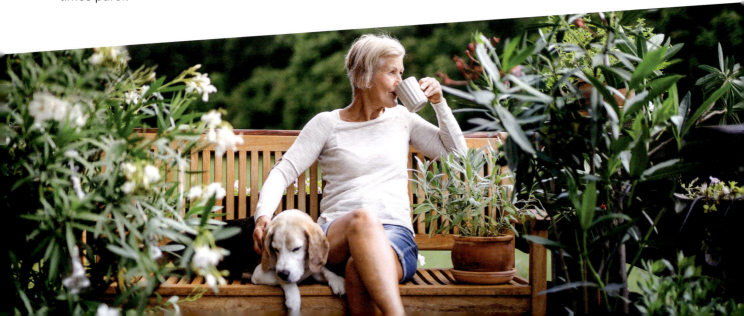

IN YOUR OWN WORDS

WHAT ARE YOUR FEELINGS AS YOU READ DESCRIPTIONS OF THE NEW EARTH?

....

....

....

Because Jesus redeemed humanity on the cross, we are invited to spend all eternity with Him in this new paradise. Until that day, God wants us to enjoy and take care of our environment.

"For you who revere My name, the sun of righteousness will rise with healing in its wings. And you will go out and leap like calves released from the stall." Malachi 4:2

Examples of goals for environment:

My goal is to spend at least 20 minutes outside at least five days a week, enjoying the health-giving benefits of the environment.

My goal is to add and sustain at least four potted plants into my home and workspace.

My goal is to begin recycling plastic, glass and cans at home within one month's time.

My goal is to add or make more accessible three things to my personal environment that I love to touch.

My goal is to declutter and organize one room in my house each month for the next six months.

LIFE APPLICATION

Take a moment to reflect on this CREATION Life study on environment.

WHAT PRINCIPLES HAVE YOU LEARNED THAT YOU WANT TO APPLY IN YOUR LIFE?

....

....

....

....

NOW, CREATE A PERSONAL GOAL FOR YOUR ENVIRONMENT.

....

....

....

....

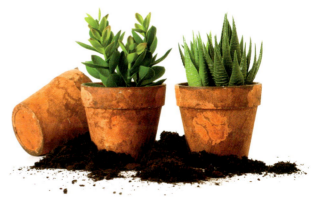

SMALL GROUP DISCUSSION QUESTIONS

1. WHICH OF THE BIBLE TEXTS ON ENVIRONMENT IMPACTED YOU MOST?

....

....

....

2. ANNIE DILLARD DESCRIBES A MOCKINGBIRD TAKING "A SINGLE STEP" OFF A ROOFTOP —
    AND IT FILLED HER WITH WONDER. WHAT IS ONE EXPERIENCE WITH NATURE THAT
    CAUSED YOU TO BE FILLED WITH WONDER?

....

....

....

3. HAVE YOU EVER BEEN — MUCH AS THE SUBMARINE CREW MEMBERS OR THE PACE TRAVELERS
    DESCRIBED — DEPRIVED OF NATURE UNTIL YOU CRAVED IT? SHARE WHAT HAPPENED.

....

....

....

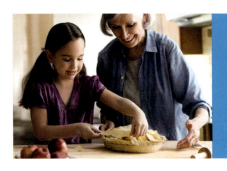

If you wish to make an apple pie from scratch, you must first invent the universe. Carl Sagan

4. WHAT DO YOU THINK IS OUR PLANET'S MOST PRESSING ENVIRONMENTAL PROBLEM? DO YOU AGREE THAT "ENVIRONMENTALISM SHOULD BE ESPECIALLY IMPORTANT TO CHRISTIANS?" WHAT GETS IN THE WAY?

....
....
....

5. WHICH OF THE FIVE SENSES MADE THE GREATEST IMPACT ON YOU?

....
....
....

6. WHICH "NATURAL HEALTH ENHANCER" DO YOU THINK YOU COULD USE MORE OF RIGHT NOW?

....
....
....

7. SHARE ONE PERSONAL GOAL WITH THE GROUP. HOW COULD THE GROUP HELP YOU REACH THIS GOAL?

....
....
....

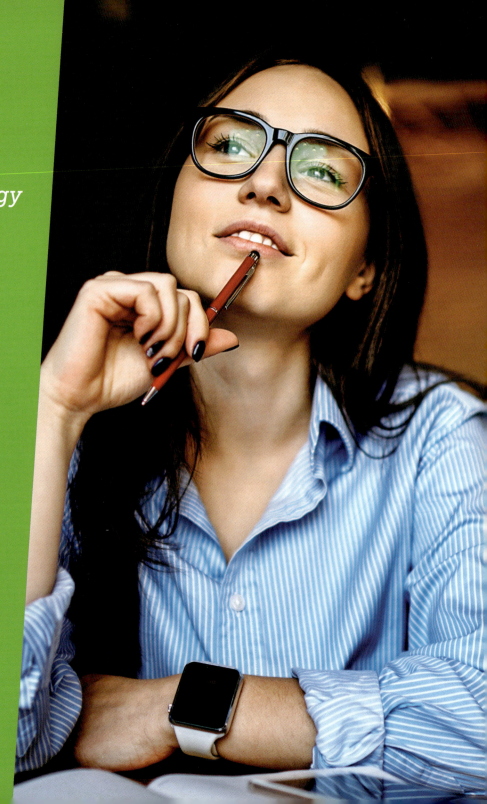

No amount of energy will ever take the place of thought.

Henry Van Dyke

ACTIVITY

Whatever you do, do it heartily,
as to the Lord and not to men. *Colossians 3:23*

MENTAL ACTIVITY

When Ben Carson was in fifth grade, he thought he was the dumbest kid in his class. Sonya Carson, his mother, had other ideas.

"You're just not living up to your potential," she said. "You have to use that good brain that God gave you, Bennie."

As a single parent, Ben's mother prayed to God for wisdom in how to raise her two sons. She received her answer and quickly shared it with Ben and his brother. "Boys, you're wasting too much of your time in front of that television. You don't get an education from staring at television all the time," she observed. "The Lord's told me what to do. So from now on, you will not watch television, except for two preselected programs each week."

"Just *two* programs?" Ben could hardly believe what his mother was saying. But she wasn't through yet.

"And *only* after you've done your homework," she added. "And that isn't all. You also have to read two books from the library each week. Every single week."

"Two books? *Two?*" Ben had never read an entire book in his life. He wasn't sure if he could even do it. But something happened the more Ben Carson read those books. He discovered how much he loved reading.

From then on, Ben Carson could not read enough. His thirst for knowledge grew until it was unquenchable. By the middle of sixth grade, he had moved to the top of the class. He also began to read the book of Proverbs everyday for wisdom.

Years later, the boy who once thought he was the dumbest kid in his fifth-grade class became Dr. Ben Carson, one of the most celebrated neurosurgeons in the world. He made medical history in 1987 as the first doctor to successfully separate conjoined twins. In 2008 he was awarded the Presidential Medal of Freedom.[1]

Living abundantly involves participating in both mental and physical activity. The mind and body are connected in countless ways, so we achieve the best performance when we learn how to use both. Mental activities such as reading, playing a musical instrument and doing crossword puzzles help to hone our minds in the same way physical exercise conditions our bodies.

Where I Am *(Place a mark on the line to show what you're feeling right now.)*

I often feel
mentally sluggish.

I'm usually clear-minded
and loving.

"The fear of the Lord is the beginning of wisdom; a good understanding have all those who do His commandments. His praise endures forever."
Psalm 111:10

The book of Proverbs often says "the fear of the Lord" is the start of wisdom. But really, what does it mean to "fear God"? Especially when elsewhere in the Bible we are told:

"There is no fear in love; but perfect love casts out fear, because fear involves torment. But he who fears has not been made perfect in love."
1 John 4:18

In the Old Testament, the word "fear" depicts an emotion not of dread and terror but rather reverence, awe and admiration. This positive quality is not about feeling panicky or scared. It's a loving, respectful response to a compassionate, wise Parent.

HOW DO WE RECEIVE GOD'S DIRECTION?

1. BE HUMBLE.

"The fear of the Lord is instruction in wisdom, and humility comes before honor."
Proverbs 15:33

Often, we don't perceive our true, needy condition because an attitude of pride and self-centeredness flows through our veins. We think, *do I really need God? Aren't I a good enough person on my own?"* What we don't realize is that we have a huge problem. Our feeble attempts at "being good" could never begin to reach God's perfect character. As the Bible describes it, "All our righteous deeds are like a polluted garment" (Isaiah 64:6). The deficit is too great, and trying to bail ourselves out is like writing a check to cover a checking overdraft fee.

Pride was the first sin. God must reject pride because it separates us from His love. We arrogantly think we know what's best for our lives and so we ignore His pleas and commands, not realizing they were given to help us live freely and fully.

One of the reasons for Christ's sacrifice on the cross was to make us humble, thus teachable. True humility recognizes reality — that without God we are nothing. In *Hope Has Its Reasons*, Becky Pippert details her journey toward healthy humility.

> Slowly I started acknowledging my own faults. I began to deal with the root problems in my life and not merely the symptoms. I saw that my pride and self-centeredness lay deep within, far deeper than I had ever imagined.
>
> And I made an exciting discovery. The more I faced myself — my self-deceptions, pockets of unbelief, false confidence, controlling devices and so on — the more I found freedom.

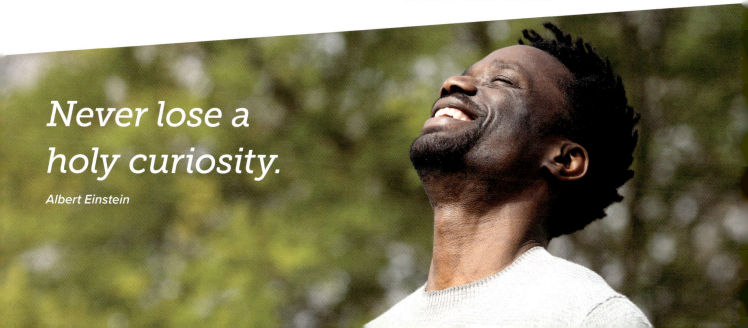

Never lose a holy curiosity.

Albert Einstein

"Thus says the Lord: 'Let not the wise man glory in his wisdom, let not the mighty man glory in his might, nor let the rich man glory in his riches; but let him who glories glory in this, that he understands and knows Me, that I am the Lord, exercising loving kindness, judgment, and righteousness in the earth, for in these I delight,' says the Lord." Jeremiah 9:23, 24

When we choose to acknowledge God's sovereignty in all things we have begun the humbling process. We are the invention; God is our Inventor. Let us draw near with humility.

"When pride comes, then comes shame; but with the humble is wisdom" Proverbs 11:2

Fortunately, if we do not presently harbor a humble spirit, we can ask God to help us.

The story is told of a proud preacher who reveled in reciting lengthy prayers to his congregation. On one occasion, he went on for an extended time. His church members fidgeted in their pews as the preacher took great pleasure in showing off his theological knowledge and vast vocabulary. Finally, the preacher finished with the words, "And, dear Lord, please help keep us humble."

Feeling pleased with himself, the preacher made his way back to his seat when he suddenly tripped on a step and fell face down in front of the congregation.

A saintly elder helped him up. "Oh, thank God!" the elder said. "Thank God for such a quick answer!"

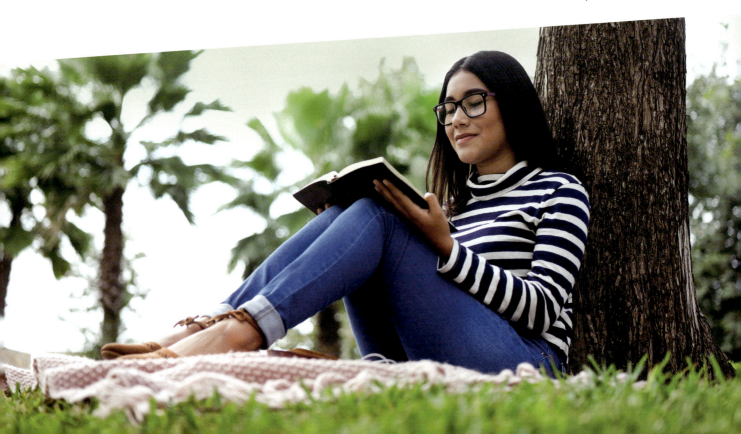

2. SEEK WISDOM.

"I love those who love Me, and those who seek Me diligently will find Me." Proverbs 8:17

God's power will give you victory over any addiction — alcohol, cigarettes, food, promiscuity, gossip, entertainment. But you must first seek wisdom. This means seeing God as greater than anything else in this world.

"And you will seek Me and find Me, when you search for Me with all your heart." Jeremiah 29:13

Start by staying consistent in your Bible study and prayer time with Him. God wants to show you how you can restore your strained relationships, whether with your mother or father, brother or sister or a longtime friend. He wants you to live a CREATION Life in every way. Look at these ideas for seeking wisdom from God daily:

We can seek wisdom through prayer.

"If any of you lacks wisdom, let him ask of God, who gives to all liberally and without reproach, and it will be given to him." James 1:5

We can seek it in the Bible and through music.

"Let the word of Christ dwell in you richly in all wisdom, teaching and admonishing one another in psalms and hymns and spiritual songs, singing with grace in your hearts to the Lord." Colossians 3:16

We can seek it through the counsel of others.

"Without counsel, plans go awry, but in the multitude of counselors they are established." Proverbs 15:22

We can seek it with assurance, trusting that God's ways are best.

"But let him ask in faith, with no doubting." James 1:6

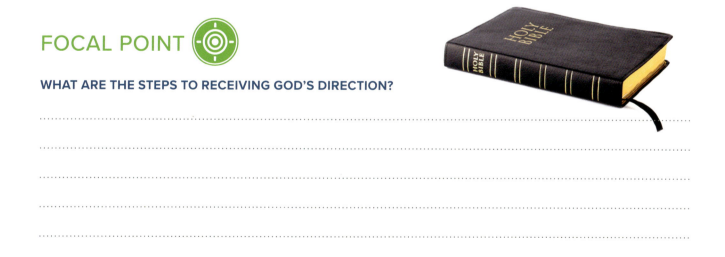

FOCAL POINT

WHAT ARE THE STEPS TO RECEIVING GOD'S DIRECTION?

....

....

....

....

....

WHAT'S THE DIFFERENCE BETWEEN KNOWLEDGE, UNDERSTANDING AND WISDOM?

KNOWLEDGE IS THE FACTS.

Those with *knowledge* are able to collect, remember and access information. They "know" the Scriptures because God's word is in them, literally. At the same time, just because we know something doesn't mean we have applied it to our lives. Many people know they should eat a healthy diet but that doesn't keep them from consistently stopping at drive-thrus.

UNDERSTANDING IS LIFTING MEANING OUT OF THE FACTS.

Those with *understanding* are able to extract meaning out of information. They "see through" the facts to the dynamics of what, how and why. Understanding is a lens that brings facts into crisp focus. Understanding produces principles. Our principles define who we are and what we believe.

WISDOM IS KNOWING WHAT TO DO NEXT.

Those with *wisdom* know which principle to apply now. Wisdom, in this sense, is the aim, and knowledge and understanding have eternal value only when guided by the wisdom of God.

When wisdom enters your heart, and knowledge is pleasant to your soul, discretion will preserve you; understanding will keep you. Proverbs 2:10, 11

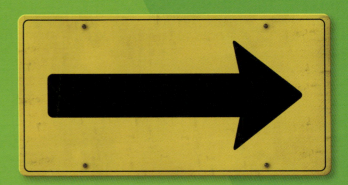

From the time He was in the temple at 12 until He began His public ministry at age 30, Jesus grew in wisdom (mentally), stature (physically) and in favor with God (spiritually) and people (socially). Jesus is the standard of balanced activity.

"My people are destroyed for lack of knowledge."
Hosea 4:6

Will Rogers quipped, "Everyone is ignorant, only on different subjects." If we do not currently have the wisdom of how to live a CREATION Life, this may prevent us from enjoying vitality. But, thank God, with the principles He so graciously gave us we can live life well — discerning, diligent and delightful.

"Do not be conformed to this world, but be transformed by the renewing of your mind, that you may prove what is that good and acceptable and perfect will of God."
Romans 12:2

"For God has not given us a spirit of fear, but of power and of love and of a sound mind."
2 Timothy 1:7

And Jesus increased in wisdom and stature, and in favor with God and men.

Luke 2:52

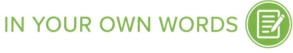

IN YOUR OWN WORDS

REWRITE THESE FOUR TEXTS AS THEY RELATE TO YOUR LIFE.

....
....
....
....
....
....
....

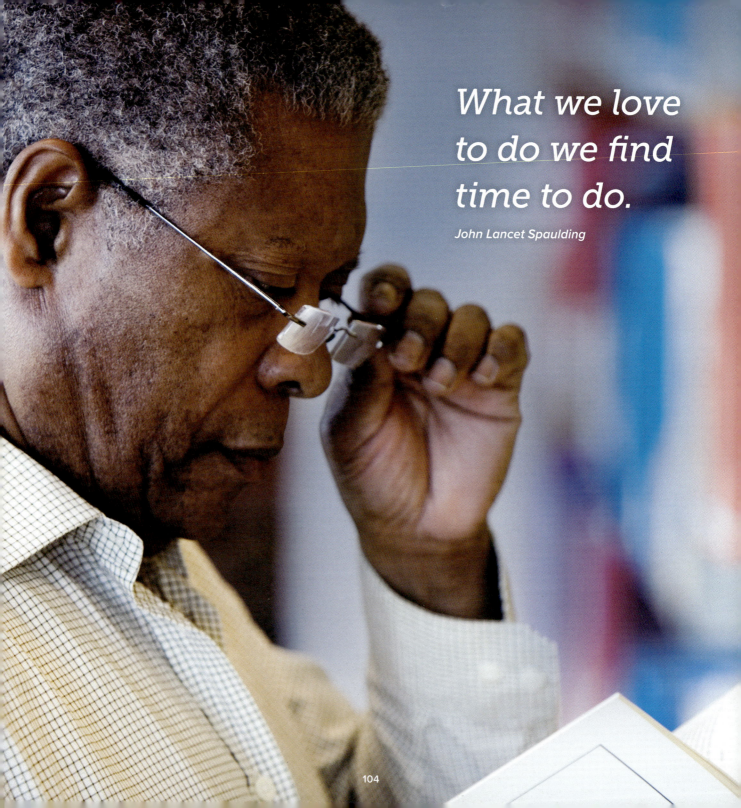

What we love to do we find time to do.

John Lancet Spaulding

"'Come now, and let us reason together,'
says the Lord." Isaiah 1:18

Just as we need to increase our knowledge, we also need to actively work on improving our ability to reason. Read a book or take a class on logic, philosophy, debate or classic reasoning. Meet regularly with a group of friends and engage in stimulating and constructive discussions. Examine all sides of each issue honestly. The more we practice these critical thinking skills, the better we will become at making good choices.

Research has determined when we don't use our brain cells they actually decrease in number. The great news is that research has also found when we *do* use our minds they grow. The adult brain can actually grow in response to regular demands placed on it, something that until recently was thought to be impossible.

Winnie the Pooh asked, "Did you ever stop to think, and forget to start again?" Exercising the brain is much like exercising the body. In fact, mental activity can actually change the physical structure of our brains. In one study, London taxi drivers were given MRIs to measure their brain's capacity for memory. The results showed significantly more hippocampal gray matter than usual. In other words, the area of the brain involved in memory was enlarged in people who used this part of their brain extensively on a daily basis.[2]

"Cleanse your hands, you sinners; and purify your
hearts, you double-minded." James 4:8

This is a call to ethical thinking — not to be hypocrites or "double-minded." When we exercise our ethical minds, we think, speak and do right. This exercise transforms us and carries with it what it means to have "the mind of Christ" (Philippians 2:4,5).

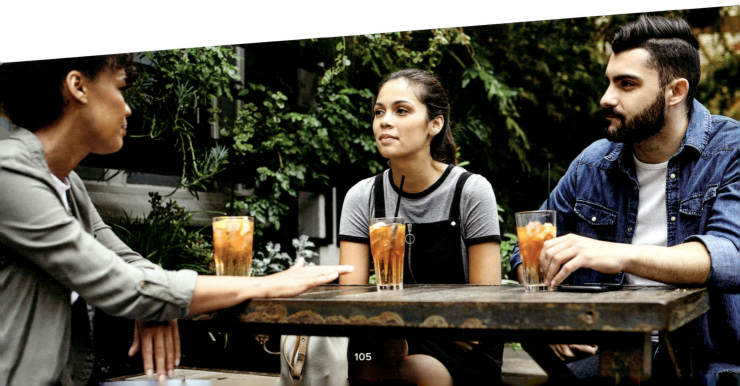

HOW CAN WE MAXIMIZE OUR MENTAL ACTIVITY?

One important time for brain function is in the morning. To sustain regular, effective mental activity you must give your brain the fuel it needs to be active. In 1995, the Pediatrics Department at the University of California at Davis hosted a group of psychologists, neuroscientists, nutritionists and physiologists to review the scientific research on breakfast. The researchers concluded the "eating of breakfast is important in learning, memory and physical well-being in both children and adults."[3]

"In a dream, in a vision of the night, when deep sleep falls upon men, while slumbering on their beds, then He opens the ears of men, and seals their instruction." Job 33:15, 16

Amazingly, we now know scientifically that during our sleep the brain is busy sorting thoughts and storing them away. Sleep allows us to "seal" what we have learned in our minds. God made our bodies to sleep at night when it is dark; this helps us to experience healthy circadian rhythms.

Researchers discovered significant association with earlier bedtimes, longer sleep length and the performance of the brain. The benefits of getting adequate sleep at the right time have been demonstrated through higher scores on exams and better overall academic performance.

Consider when you feel mentally slow and lethargic. It's often when you're sleep-deprived. Adequate sleep enables the brain to operate at peak levels.

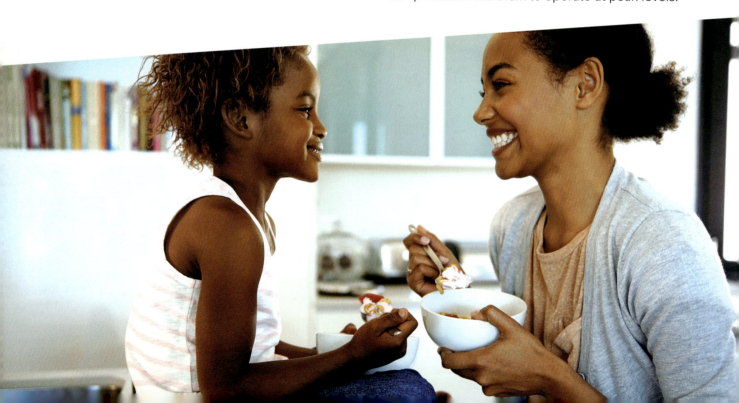

LIFE APPLICATION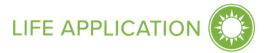

Take a moment to reflect on this CREATION Life emphasis on mental activity.

WHAT PRINCIPLES HAVE YOU LEARNED THAT YOU WANT TO APPLY IN YOUR LIFE?

....

....

....

....

....

....

....

NOW, CREATE A PERSONAL GOAL FOR YOUR MENTAL ACTIVITY.

....

....

....

....

....

....

....

Examples of goals for mental activity:

My goal is to take one issue each day and spend ten minutes writing down every conceivable point of view on the topic.

My goal is to start a hobby such as crossword puzzles, Sudoku, word games, chess or logic problems that will sharpen my mental skills.

My goal is to earnestly and humbly ask for God's wisdom in the pressing matters of my life. By daily praying for it, reading God's Word and acting on what God reveals to me, I trust God will grant me His wisdom.

My goal is to memorize and share with another person one Bible text each week.

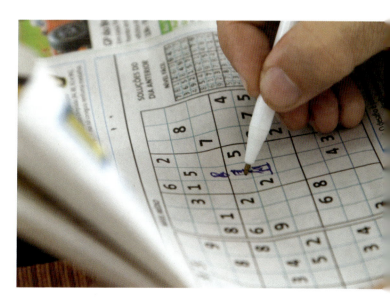

PHYSICAL ACTIVITY

An intimate connection between mental and physical activity exists. At some point, a healthy person enters the physical realm. As the saying goes, "You cannot plow a field by turning it over in your mind."

Upon arriving at her sixth decade of life, Hulda Crooks decided to become serious about physical activity. She was overweight and out of shape, so much so that the only exercise she could manage was to walk around her yard. Day by day she began to increase the distance. Soon she could make it around her block, and then her neighborhood.

At the age of 66, she climbed Mt. Whitney, the tallest mountain in the lower 48 United States (14,494 feet). By 90, she had climbed it annually 22 times (missing twice because of bad weather) and was still going strong. She was the oldest person to reach the summit. To top it off, she later climbed Mt. Fuji in Japan. A fitness evaluation showed she had the cardiovascular fitness level of a person at least 30 years younger.

"And the Lord God formed man of the dust of the ground, and breathed into his nostrils the breath of life; and man became a living being." Genesis 2:7

God's breath gave life, including spiritual, mental and physical life. These parts are inseparable and fully dependent on one another. Yet some believe that physical life is somehow flawed and inferior to the other realms. This line of thinking originated with the Greeks, who taught the spiritual realm was far superior to the physical.

Richard J. Foster comments, "I do not have a spirit: I am a spirit. Likewise, I do not have a body: I am a body." The spirit spoken of in the Bible is God's indwelling Spirit.

"Do you not know that your body is the temple of the Holy Spirit who is in you, whom you have from God and you are not your own? For you were bought at a price; therefore glorify God in your body and in your spirit, which are God's." 1 Corinthians 6:19, 20

Physical activity helps the body function optimally, reduces stress and enables us to better hear the voice of God. Activity helps the brain to think clearly and comprehend spiritual truths. Believe it or not, physical fitness can enhance our spiritual walk.

Where I Am *(Place a mark on the line to show what you're feeling right now.)*

I generally feel physically unfit.   **I feel physically vibrant and strong.**

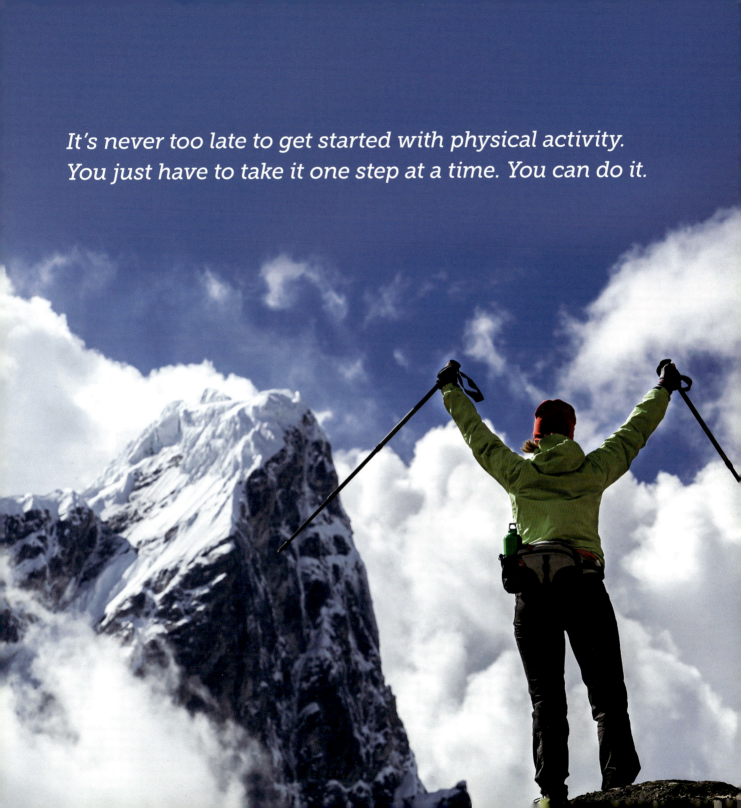

It's never too late to get started with physical activity. You just have to take it one step at a time. You can do it.

IN YOUR OWN WORDS

WHAT DO YOU SEE AS THE CONNECTION BETWEEN PHYSICAL AND SPIRITUAL HEALTH?

....

....

....

....

....

....

Now about the fourth watch of the night He came to them, walking on the sea, and would have passed them by.

Mark 6:48

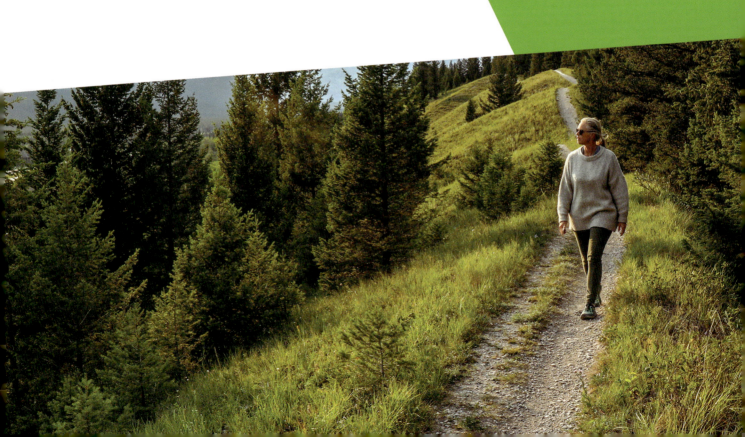

OUR ULTIMATE EXAMPLE

Today, we pay with plastic for plastic utensils and pizza delivery — anything to make our lives easier. Yet for all our modern conveniences we still feel rushed, overwhelmed and exhausted. "It is ironic," writes Jeremy Rifkin in *Time Wars,* "that in a culture so committed to saving time we feel increasingly deprived of the very thing we value." Sue Monk Kidd tags us as "quickaholics." We want food. Quickly. We want entertainment. Quickly. We want to finish reading this page. Quickly. What we really need is to slow down and experience the life God has given us on a deeper level.

The story is told of a man phoning an airline and asking, "How long does it take to fly from Montreal to Vancouver?"

"Just a minute," the clerk replied.

"Thank you," said the man, and then he hung up.

In Bible times, physical activity was a way of life. There were no automobiles or mass transit. No online shopping or mobile phones. The primary mode of transportation was simply walking.

Walking slows us down. It allows time to reflect, and incorporates muscles throughout the whole body, including the legs, back, abdominals, arms and shoulders.

"Is this not the carpenter's Son?" Matthew 13:55

As a carpenter, Jesus held a physically demanding job. He worked with a hammer, saw, plane, file and chisel. And, naturally, He walked everywhere He went.

"And Jesus, walking by the Sea of Galilee... " Matthew 4:18

"After these things Jesus walked... " John 7:1

Jesus is our best example of how to live a CREATION Life. The *Journal of the American Medical Association* published an article entitled "On the Physical Death of Jesus Christ." In the section "Health of Jesus," medical researchers from the Mayo Clinic state, "the rigors of Jesus' ministry (that is, traveling by foot throughout Palestine) would have precluded any major physical illness or weak general constitution. Accordingly, it is reasonable to assume that Jesus was in good physical condition before his walk to Gethsemane … Jesus did have a rigorous ministry."

This conclusion was confirmed by carefully looking at the places Jesus walked as recorded in the biblical account. The final assessment: When he was traveling, *Jesus walked on average 25 miles a day,* so he had to be in good physical shape!

Moreover, as He taught, His disciples walked with Him. It became a mobile school.

Today, we can still enjoy walking and talking with Him. One invigorating way is to go for a walk in nature and talk with God. Walk at a leisurely pace and pay close attention to all that you see and hear. Allow God to speak to you through the beauty of His creation.

Our God is a God of movement.

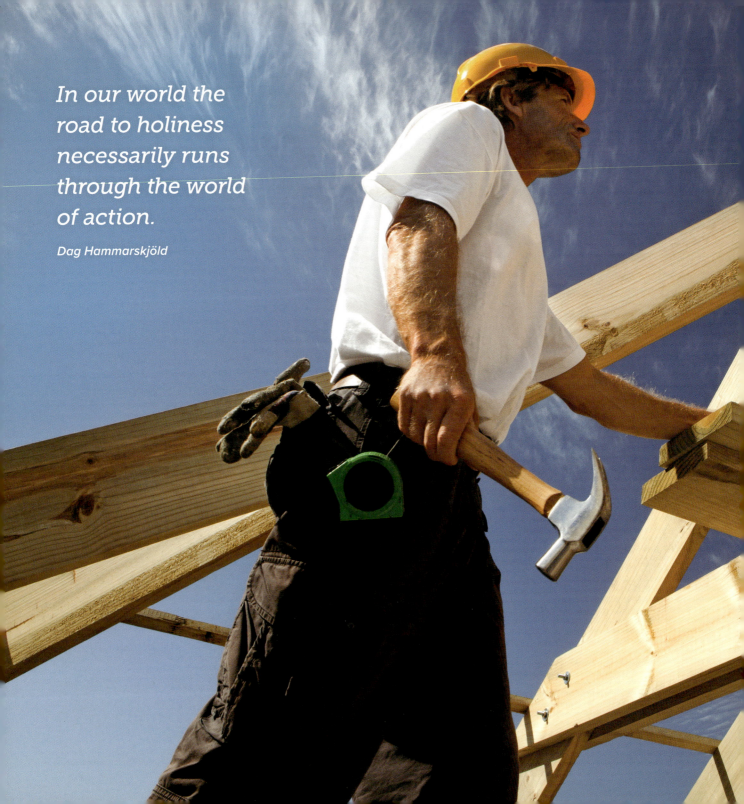

In our world the road to holiness necessarily runs through the world of action.

Dag Hammarskjöld

THE SO-THAT PRINCIPLE

Consider a light bulb. If the outer glass looks great but no light is emitted, is it a "healthy" bulb? Actually, the light bulb's health is determined by only one aspect: *whether it produces light.* That is the sole reason for its existence. Whatever prevents it from producing light makes the bulb unhealthy.

We often miss an understanding of the "so-that" principle. A light bulb exists *so that* it can shine light. So why should people be healthy? Answers to that question often include, "So I'll look better," or "So I'll have more energy." But those reasons don't go far enough. We all know people who work hard to change their outward appearance but do little to change their health on the inside. Beyond appearance and energy stands a much higher goal.

Love is the reason for human existence. Love is to people as light is to the light bulb. Whatever prevents us from loving makes us unhealthy. This love involves our minds and our bodies. *Everything we do should be done so that we can love better* — whether eating organically, praying, running errands or listening to music. Love is the supreme goal of life. Ultimately nothing else matters because nothing else lasts.

"Though I speak with the tongues of men and of angels, but have not love, I have become sounding brass or a clanging cymbal. And though I have the gift of prophecy, and understand all mysteries and all knowledge, and though I have all faith, so that I could remove mountains, but have not love, I am nothing. And though I bestow all my goods to feed the poor, and though I give my body to be burned, but have not love, it profits me nothing."
1 Corinthians 13:1-3

The highest form of love is loving God. Unless we are in love with God, we are not fully alive; we are sleepwalking through a near-life experience, settling for blurred, dim days and experiences that can never satisfy our longings. But that's not what Jesus desires for us.

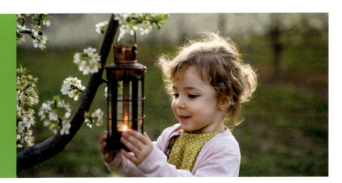

God is light and in Him is no darkness at all.

John 1:15

STRENGTH TRAINING

"God is our refuge and strength, a very present help in trouble." Psalm 46:1

At our weakest moments, we may feel comforted by the fact that we serve a compassionate God. Strength comes through quiet confidence. The more we learn to trust and rely on Him, the more He will strengthen us.

"For thus says the Lord God, the Holy One of Israel: 'In returning and rest you shall be saved; in quietness and confidence shall be your strength.'" Isaiah 30:15

While Jesus was praying in the Garden of Gethsemane, right before they took Him away to be tried and suffer death in our place, God the Father sent help to strengthen Him.

"Then an angel appeared to Him from heaven, strengthening Him." Luke 22:43

Not only is God all-powerful, He makes His power available to us.

"'So we built the wall, and the entire wall was joined together up to half its height, for the people had a mind to work.'" Nehemiah 4:6

Having "a mind to work" means cooperating with God. Many times, when Jesus healed people He asked them to do something to demonstrate their faith. Christ expects us to cooperate with Him in our healing and growth.

"Now a certain man was there who had an infirmity thirty-eight years. When Jesus saw him lying there, and knew that he already had been in that condition a long time, He said to him, "Do you want to be made well?" The sick man answered Him, "Sir, I have no man to put me into the pool when the water is stirred up; but while I am coming, another steps down before me." Jesus said to him, "Rise, take up your bed and walk." And immediately the man was made well, took up his bed, and walked." John 5:5-9

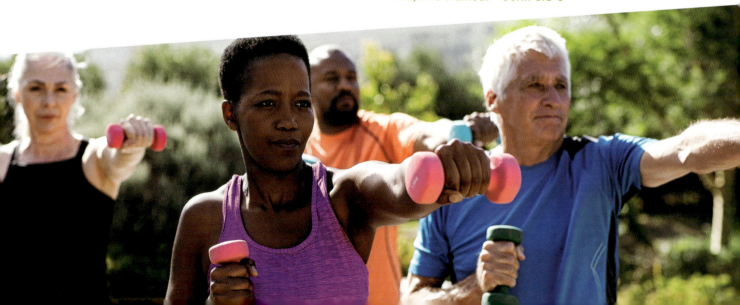

IN YOUR OWN WORDS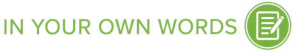

IN WHAT AREAS OF YOUR LIFE DO YOU NEED GOD TO PROVIDE YOU WITH STRENGTH?

....

....

....

....

....

....

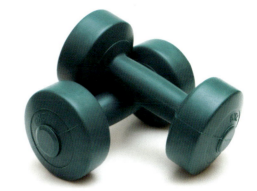

One woman started regularly participating in aerobic physical activity and strength training. She soon noted how her increase in physical strength was generating positive effects on the other important components of her life. She was "stronger" in her job with her co-workers — she now possessed the energy to tactfully and confidently stand up for what was right.

Large research studies have shown benefits for people that are physically active. These benefits include being happier and having less depression, fewer strokes, lower risk of hip fractures and stronger immune systems. Active people are also less likely to catch a cold or the flu, and they live longer. With such great benefits available to us, we must seriously ask ourselves, "What's stopping me from being more active?"

Centuries before the jogging trend was launched, running illustrations were used in Scripture.

"Therefore we also, since we are surrounded by so great a cloud of witnesses, let us lay aside every weight, and the sin which so easily ensnares us, and let us run with endurance the race that is set before us. Hebrews 12:1

"Do you not know that those who run in a race all run, but one receives the prize? Run in such a way that you may obtain it." 1 Corinthians 9:24

In this race of life, physical activity helps us to run and finish strong. As we regulate our bodies toward becoming more active we'll find greater discipline in other areas of our lives.

MORNING ACTIVITY

While getting physical activity at other times of the day is definitely beneficial, morning physical activity does carry its advantages.

First, it has been found that more than 90 percent of those who exercise "consistently" exercise in the morning. Think about it: many times unexpected events arise and push activity by the wayside. Morning physical activity helps us to be more persistent.

Second, physical activity in the morning "jump starts" your metabolism and keeps it elevated throughout the day. If you choose to be physically active at night you'll miss out on much of the benefits of your elevated metabolism.

Third, exercising in the morning gives you the satisfaction of knowing that you have already gotten in your activity for the day. You don't have to worry about trying to fit it in if something unexpected comes up.

Fourth, physical activity helps you to be mentally alert. Think of the benefit of being more mentally awake all day — not just a few hours.

With physical activity, sometimes we carry an all-or-none mentality. We often think if we don't get the activity we want just when we want it, then it's not worth it. But research shows that an accumulation of just three 10-minute sessions a day can make a tremendous impact on our health. Every minute helps.

So many of us long for balance in our lives, but our lives will never be truly balanced until we make activity a vital part of our day. And, in the end, we don't want to merely do "our best" — we want to do our *balanced* best.

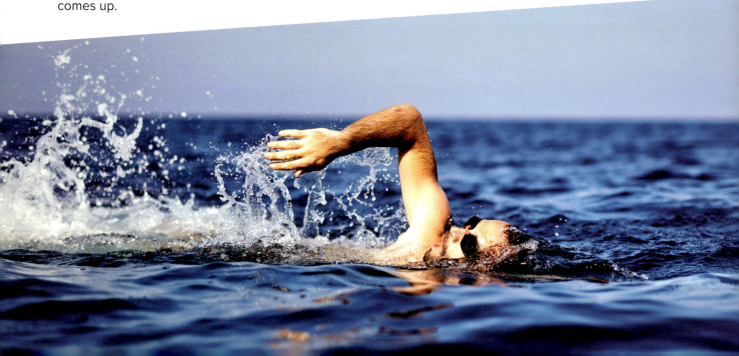

TO OBTAIN OPTIMAL RESULTS FROM PHYSICAL ACTIVITY:

- Find an activity or two you like; then vary it day to day so you don't get bored doing the same thing.

- Invest in good shoes and comfortable clothing.

- Exercise with a friend — you're more likely to do the activity if someone helps keep you accountable.

- Try to get outside to take advantage of the health benefits of fresh air and sunshine.

- Remember, no activity is too small. Mild and moderate activities such as walking or gardening show numerous health benefits.

- Strength training is another important component and can help you lose weight.

- To receive added benefits, participate in physical activity in the morning.

- Exercise at least three days a week with vigorous activity and at least five days a week if you are doing moderate physical activity.

- For even better results, include interval training and intermittent training, which includes resting. And remember, you can participate in as short as three 10-minute sessions for a total of 30 minutes a day and still gain great results.

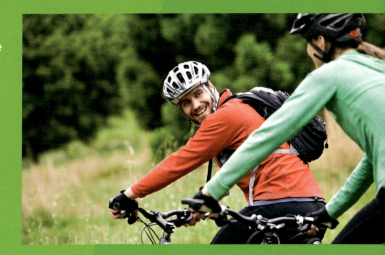

The world is full of willing people, some willing to work, the others willing to let them.

Robert Frost

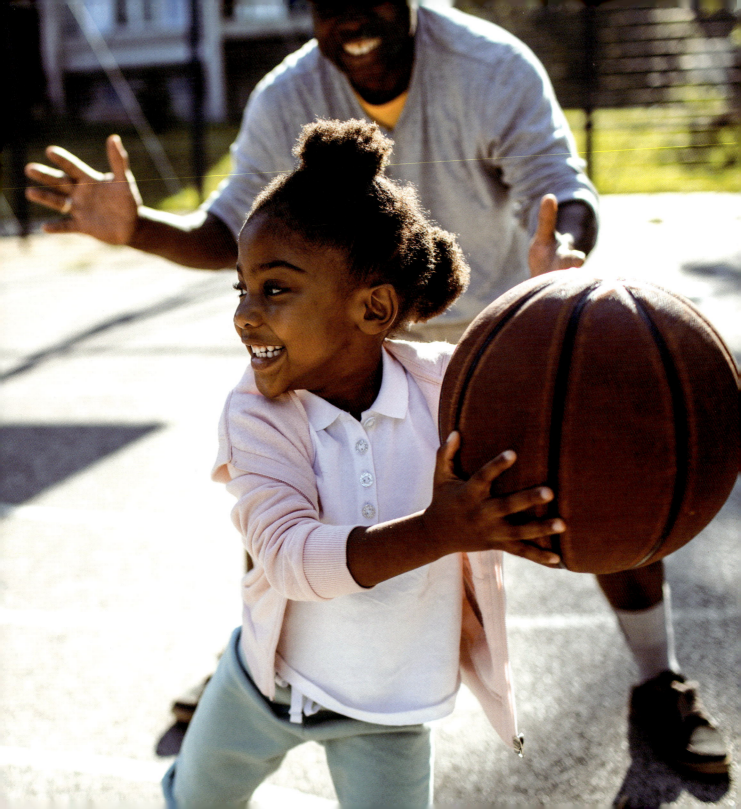

LIFE APPLICATION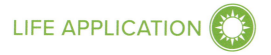

Take a moment to reflect on this CREATION Life emphasis on physical activity.

WHAT PRINCIPLES HAVE YOU LEARNED THAT YOU WANT TO APPLY IN YOUR LIFE?

....

....

....

....

....

....

....

NOW, CREATE A PERSONAL GOAL FOR YOUR PHYSICAL ACTIVITY.

....

....

....

....

....

....

....

....

Examples of goals for physical activity:

My goal is to participate in a strength-training program that involves each of the major muscle groups two times a week.

My goal is to play/exercise with the kids for at least 15 minutes five days of the week.

My goal is to walk and talk with God in prayer 30 minutes in the morning at least three days each week.

My goal is to walk for 10 minutes in the morning before breakfast, and then after two of the three meals of the day on at least six days per week, for a total of 30 minutes of exercise on those days.

Idle folks have the least leisure.

John Ray

SMALL GROUP DISCUSSION QUESTIONS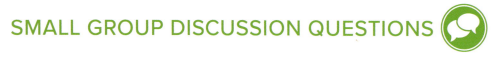

1. **WHAT BIBLE TEXT ON ACTIVITY INSPIRED YOU MOST?**

....

....

....

2. **DO YOU REALLY THINK SLEEPING WELL AND EATING A GOOD BREAKFAST WILL HELP YOUR MIND?**

....

....

....

3. **HAVE YOU MADE A DECISION ABOUT ONE ASPECT OF MENTAL ACTIVITY THAT YOU PLAN TO BEGIN? PLEASE SHARE WITH THE GROUP.**

....

....

....

4. **WHERE COULD YOU USE SOME WISDOM IN YOUR LIFE RIGHT NOW?**

....

....

....

5. HOW CAN YOU APPLY THE "SO-THAT PRINCIPLE" TO YOUR LIFE?

....

....

....

6. "JESUS WALKED." HOW SHOULD THIS SIMPLE TRUTH AFFECT US TODAY?

....

....

....

7. WHAT'S YOUR GOAL FOR PHYSICAL ACTIVITY? HOW CAN OUR GROUP HELP YOU REACH THIS GOAL?

....

....

....

He who cannot find time for exercise must sooner or later find time for illness.

Benjamin Franklin

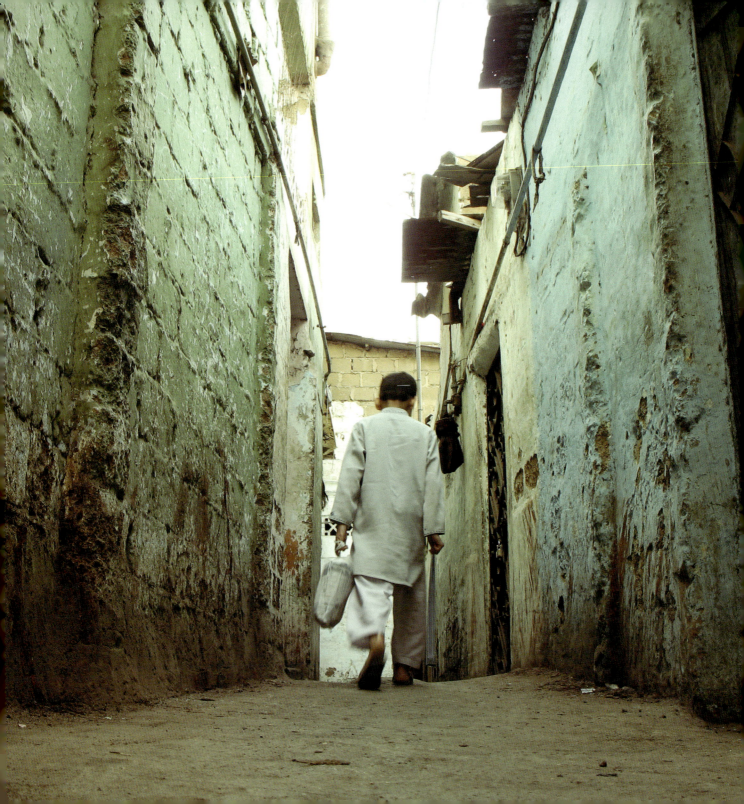

TRUST IN GOD

Trust in the Lord with all your heart,
and lean not on your own understanding;
in all your ways acknowledge Him,
And He shall direct your paths. *Proverbs 3:5, 6*

A trusting friendship with God is vital if we are ever to achieve the fullness of CREATION Life. The question is: Can God truly be trusted? What sort of friendship does He offer?

Canon Goldsmith was a missionary for the Anglican Church in India. One day, he entrusted a large sum of money to his servant and told him to buy supplies. Instead, the servant took the money and disappeared. Canon was upset, but not for the typical reasons. We pick up the story after he decided to use any means necessary to find the servant.

> For days he searched for the man. Finally finding him, in deep humility he said, "I am so sorry I paid you such small wages for your work that you had to do a thing like this. Come back and keep working for me and I will give you better pay."

> The servant was completely overcome by this expression of love and confidence. He went back, thoroughly repented, and became Canon Goldsmith's devoted and trusted servant, friend and brother for life.[1]

Canon's loyalty to his servant was not affected by how loyal his servant was to him. He determined to love no matter what.

This interaction is a beautiful example of God's gracious love for all people. God desires a relationship with us regardless of our mistakes. Let's explore the ways we know we can trust Him.

DOES GOD WANT A FRIENDSHIP?

"Yes, I have loved you with an everlasting love; therefore with loving kindness I have drawn you."
Jeremiah 31:3

"How often I wanted to gather your children together, as a hen gathers her brood under her wings."
Luke 13:34

"No longer do I call you servants, for a servant does not know what his master is doing; but I have called you friends." *John 15:15*

As revealed in these texts, there is no doubt of God's deep yearning. He greatly desires a friendship with us, but for that to occur we must trust Him.

In his book *Mere Christianity*, C. S. Lewis describes where the battle for trusting God starts:

> It comes the very moment you wake up each morning. All your wishes and hopes for the day rush at you like wild animals. And the first job each morning consists simply in shoving them all back; in listening to that other voice, taking that other point of view, letting that other larger, stronger, quieter life come flowing in. And so on, all day. Standing back from all your natural fussings and frettings; coming in out of the wind.

Trust is also like a living tree. The deeper we are rooted in Jesus, the more this connection helps our trust to grow.

"Blessed are those who trust in the Lord, whose trust is the Lord. They shall be like a tree planted by water, sending out its roots by the stream. It shall not fear when heat comes, and its leaves shall stay green; in the year of drought it is not anxious, and it does not cease to bear fruit." *Jeremiah 17:7, 8*

As the branches of a tree provide cool shade from the hot sun, trust serves as a covering that keeps us calm and secure.

Where I Am *(Place a mark on the line to show what you're feeling right now.)*

**I don't trust anyone, really.
Not even God.**

**I trust God with absolutely
everything in my life.**

RIGHTEOUSNESS BY TRUST

Note how Romans chapter 5, verses 1 and 2 is translated, first by the New King James Version.

"Therefore, having been justified by faith, we have peace with God through our Lord Jesus Christ, through whom also we have access by faith into this grace in which we stand."

Now, contrast that with the Jewish New Testament translation by David H. Stern.

"So, since we have come to be considered righteous by God because of our trust, let us continue to have shalom with God through our Lord, Yeshua the Messiah. Also through him and on the ground of our trust, we have gained access to this grace in which we stand."

Reducing the texts to their bare essentials, we find a simple formula: **FAITH = TRUST**

That's what faith is, after all. Our trust in Jesus gives us access to God's amazing grace. God justifies us when we trust in the finished work of Jesus. We enjoy "righteousness by trust."

FOCAL POINT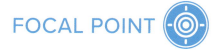

Try substituting the word "trust" whenever you use "faith." The result for many is discovering life in wholehearted, peaceful dependence.

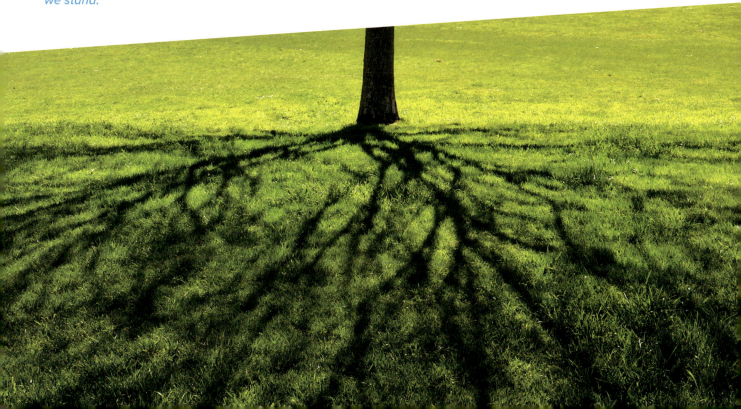

CAN WE TRUST GOD TO KEEP HIS PROMISES?

Two children, Sam and Gretchen, were talking about what they had learned so far in life.

Gretchen said, "If you have $2, and you ask your father for $4, how much will you have?

Sam said, "Two dollars."

Gretchen stared at him. "You don't know your math."

Sam replied, "You don't know my father."

Fortunately, our heavenly Father has promised to provide us with everything we need — and to catch us when we "fall."

"And my God shall supply all your need according to His riches in glory by Christ Jesus." Philippians 4:19

"'I will restore health to you, and heal you of your wounds,' says the Lord." Jeremiah 30:17

"For all the promises of God in [Jesus] are yes, and in Him Amen." 2 Corinthians 1:20

IN YOUR OWN WORDS

PARAPHRASE THE PREVIOUS THREE TEXTS.

....

....

....

....

....

....

....

....

....

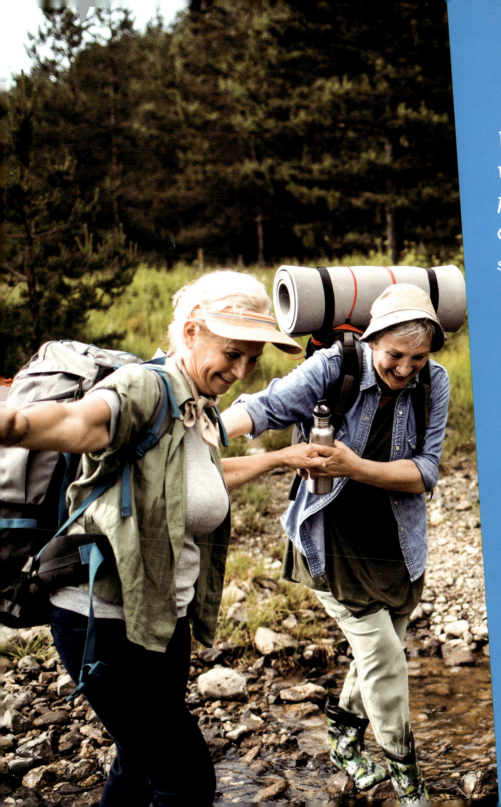

Without trust we won't achieve primary greatness or lasting success.

Stephen Covey

FEAR NOT

Learning to trust fearlessly provides tremendous benefit to our lives. With our trust placed firmly on God, we can endure anything.

"God is our refuge and strength, a very present help in trouble. Therefore we will not fear, even though the earth be removed." Psalm 46:1, 2

"Yea, though I walk through the valley of the shadow of death, I will fear no evil; for You are with me." Psalm 23:4

One constant appears in the Bible whenever God approaches humans. We see it several times in Luke's account of the birth of Jesus. As the angel approaches Mary to announce that she will bear God's Son he says to her, "Do not be afraid, Mary."

Likewise, Zechariah is startled by an angel who urges him, "Do not be afraid." Even the angel who appears to the shepherds has to comfort them: "Be not afraid."

Jesus Himself assures His followers, "Let not your hearts be troubled, neither let them be afraid." The night He walks on the water toward the disciples they are petrified. But Jesus affirms to them, "It is I. Don't be afraid." Elsewhere He comforts us with, "Fear not, little flock." After the Resurrection, an angel says to the women seeking Jesus' body, "Do not be afraid." Then Jesus appears to the hiding disciples and reassures, "Do not be afraid."

Do we get it? Just as we don't want our own children to live in fear, God doesn't want us, His children, to live in fear.

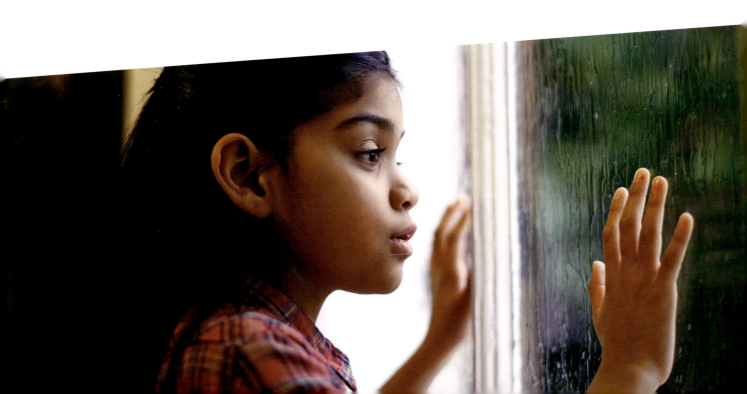

CHECK IT OUT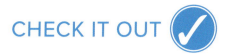

I TEND TO BE DISTRUSTING AND FEARFUL BECAUSE

- ☐ **IN THE PAST I'VE BEEN HURT AND DISAPPOINTED.**
- ☐ **I'VE SEEN TOO MANY SCARY MOVIES AND DISTURBING TV PROGRAMS.**
- ☐ **I FEEL I CAN'T BE TRUSTED.**
- ☐ **MY ENVIRONMENT IS NOT SAFE.**
- ☐ **I DON'T KNOW ANY TRUSTWORTHY ROLE-MODELS.**
- ☐ **I'M TIED IN KNOTS AND TIRED MOST OF THE TIME.**
- ☐

NOTE TO READER: Now <u>underline</u> and **star** ✷ words
in these Bible texts that will help you live a more trusting lifestyle.

*"I sought the Lord, and He heard me, and delivered me
from all my fears." Psalm 34:4*

*"And He said to me, 'My grace is sufficient for you,
for My strength is made perfect in weakness.'*
2 Corinthians 12:9

*"No temptation has overtaken you except such as is
common to man; but God is faithful, who will not allow
you to be tempted beyond what you are able, but with
the temptation will also make the way of escape, that
you may be able to bear it." 1 Corinthians 10:13*

"Whenever I am afraid, I will trust in You." Psalm 56:3

WORRY — FEAR'S CRIPPLING COUSIN

The opposite of trust is not doubt, but worry. Doubt can eventually strengthen faith as we reason through different issues, yet worry always drains us. The English word *worry* comes from the German *wurgen*, which means "to strangle, to choke." It's not hard to see how worrying chokes a person's spirit, making healthy functioning impossible. That's why Jesus cautions,

"I say to you, do not worry about your life, what you will eat or what you will drink: nor about your body, what you will put on.... But seek first the kingdom of God and His righteousness, and all these things shall be added to you. Therefore do not worry about tomorrow, for tomorrow will worry about its own things." Matthew 6:25, 33, 34

Once, for a teaching lesson, a middle-school teacher filled a large vat with five gallons of water.

"This water," he said, "represents our trust in God. Five gallons of faith." He held up a bottle of cooking oil. "This oil represents our worry." He poured in one cup of oil.

"Now, Eric," he told a student, "I want you to mix this little bit of worry into our large faith so that the worry disappears." Happy to oblige, Eric churned the water into a froth. The water continued spinning for half a minute.

At first, the oil couldn't be seen, but as the water stilled, six globules congealed on top. The globules flattened, moved toward each other and formed an oily film. In the end, one cup of worry covered five gallons of faith. Just as oil and water don't mix, worry and trust cannot coexist.

As we're stilled in bed after a spinning day, worries congeal, expand and cover our peace of mind. We must trust God entirely, giving our worries to Him. *If a problem is not large enough to be acted upon or handled with prayer, it's not big enough to worry about.*

LIFE APPLICATION

WHAT WORRIES COME TO YOUR MIND RIGHT NOW? GIVE THEM OVER TO GOD.

1. ....

....

2. ....

....

3. ....

....

Some people think the Christian life means having "blind faith." That is, we accept everything we are told and turn off our brains to any contrary evidence. This couldn't be further from the truth. As Ellen White observes, we are called to love God "with all our mind" (see Luke 10:27, 28).

God never asks us to believe, without giving sufficient evidence upon which to base our faith. His existence, His character, the truthfulness of His Word, are all established by testimony that appeals to our reason; and this testimony is abundant. Yet God has never removed the possibility of doubt. Our faith must rest upon evidence, not demonstration. Those who wish to doubt will have opportunity; while those who really desire to know the truth will find plenty of evidence upon which to rest their faith.

When the train goes through the tunnel and the world gets dark, do you jump out? Of course not. You sit still and trust the engineer to get you through.

Corrie Ten Boom

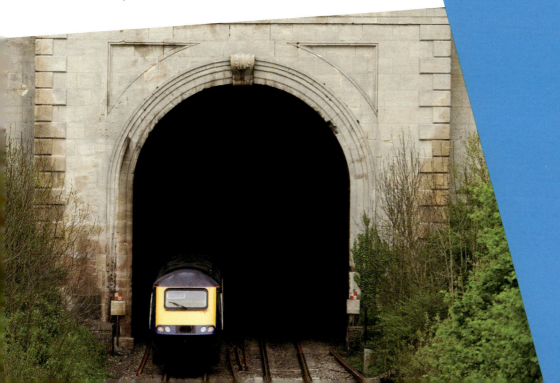

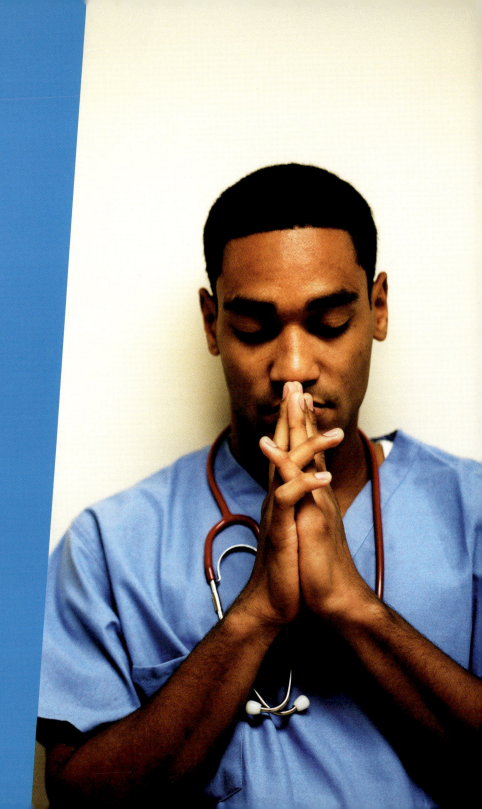

My Prayer: God, take these worries of mine and bury them beneath Your love. They are Yours, now. I do not fear tomorrow, for I know You are already there.

CAN WE BE TRUSTED?

Every solid, growing relationship is based on trust — parent-child, husband-wife, friend-friend — each healthy association in our lives sprouts from the fresh, fertile soil of trust. Can you imagine living in a "paradise" that includes untrustworthy people? It's impossible. We would be forever suspicious and fearful. A world without trust can never be paradise; it's hell instead.

"Many proclaim themselves loyal, but who can find one worthy of trust? The righteous walk in integrity — happy are the children who follow them!"
Proverbs 20:6, 7

So how does God work it out for us to be able to trust Him? He uses all the resources and attributes of the threefold Godhead. The grace of God's *Son* enables us to be humbly teachable, the unconditional love of God the *Father* equips us to be loving and the indwelling *Spirit* of God empowers us to be trustworthy.

Jesus' life and death showed the universe that God is a Friend who can always be trusted. The real question should be, *Can God trust us?* If we can't be trusted with little things here, can we be trusted with the universe ?

"He who is faithful in what is least is faithful also in much; and he who is unjust in what is least is unjust also in much." Luke 16:10

God's ability to trust us — to have faith in us — is dependent on something that's often unpopular: obedience. An old Christian hymn attests, "Trust and obey, for there's no other way." Thankfully, God gives us grace enough for both of these.

The incredible thing about living in obedience to God is how liberating it all is. We are freed to be the men and women God created us to be. The more we learn to obey Christ, the more we find authentic rest for our souls.

"Come to Me, all you who labor and are heavy laden, and I will give you rest. Take My yoke upon you and learn from Me, for I am gentle and lowly in heart, and you will find rest for your souls. For My yoke is easy and My burden is light." Matthew 11:28-30

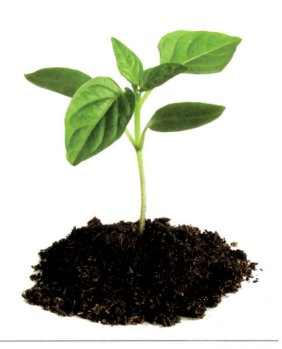

DIALOGUE IN PRAYER

Often, we labor under the illusion that prayer must be something formal, desperate or magical. Sir Eric Roll tells the story of a little boy who was overheard praying fervently, "Tokyo, Tokyo, Tokyo." Later, when he was asked why, the boy replied, "I just took my geography test in school and I've been praying to the Lord to make Tokyo the capital of France."

Our prayers aren't meant to miraculously change the world's geography. They're also not blank checks to guarantee us anything we want. When we pray, we commune with the Father and we gradually realize our total dependence on Him. Without Him, we could not even draw our next breath.

Some people ask, "what is the secret to prayer?" This implies that the answer is hidden or hard to find. It isn't, it is revealed in the Bible. The first thing to remember about prayer is that God loves you and wants to answer your prayers, just as any loving

father wants to say "yes" to his children. Second, the Bible also tells us to pray without ceasing — meaning start each day with prayer, pray often — live in a spirit of prayer. The last thing to remember is God wants us to believe He will answer our prayers — for our good. That does not mean we always get a timely answer or the one we wanted, it means God cares no matter what the outcome.

Sometimes God takes an indirect route to answer our prayers. The mother of Augustine prayed all night that God would stop her son from going to Italy because she wanted him to become a Christian. While she was praying, Augustine sailed away to Italy — where he later converted to Christianity. Naturally, his mother believed for a time that her prayers had gone unheard.

We really don't know what God is up to when He says "wait" or "no" to our prayers. That's where trust comes in.

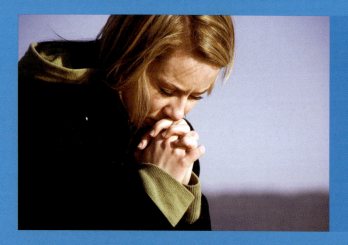

It's the cracked ones that let the light through.

Paul Moore

IN YOUR OWN WORDS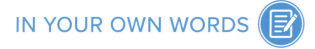

Try asking God each time you pray, "What would You have me do?" Then *focus on Jesus* and *listen* for impressions that align with His character. Hearing past internal noise requires concentrated practice. However, once you make asking and listening a habit, you will become more decisive, productive and peaceful.

"Your ears shall hear a word behind you, saying, 'This is the way, walk in it.'"   *Isaiah 30:21*

Prayer is in part a mystery. What we do know for sure is *somehow prayer enables God and ennobles us.*

When life's four worst stressors — fear, hopelessness, lack of self-worth and absence of love — threaten to devastate, we look to God for answers. Through our prayer dialogue we seek His divine leading.

GOD, WHAT WOULD YOU HAVE ME DO TODAY?

....

....

....

....

....

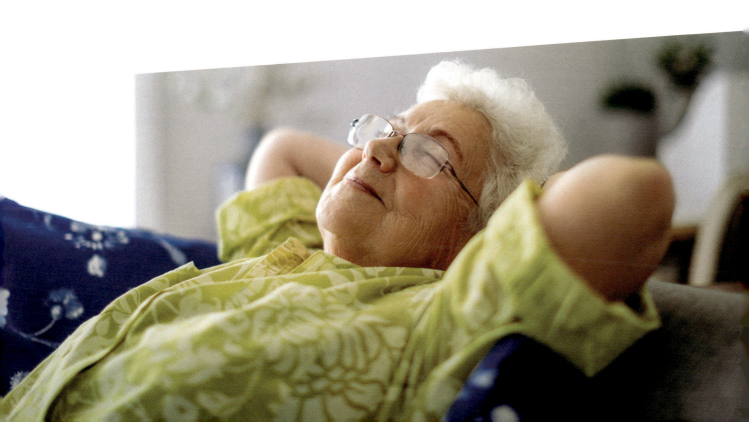

TRUST IN ACTION

Without corresponding actions, kind words are meaningless. When a person claims to love another but is abusive and violent, how genuine, really, is that love?

Sometimes trust needs to simply take action. With the Israelites trapped on the banks of the Red Sea and Pharaoh's army closing in, Moses gave a stirring speech and received a surprising response.

"And Moses said to the people, 'Do not be afraid. Stand still, and see the salvation of the Lord, which He will accomplish for you today. For the Egyptians whom you see today, you shall see again no more forever. The Lord will fight for you, and you shall hold your peace.' And the Lord said to Moses, 'Why do you cry to Me? Tell the children of Israel to go forward.'" Exodus 14:13-15

In other words, "Quit talking! You know the right course to take. Just do it." Many times, we already know what we need to do, but lack the will to do it. That's when God tells us: "Go forward. I'll be with you."

"If you know these things, blessed are you if you do them." John 13:17

An active prayer life is truly a sign of trust in action. Jesus kept His prayer connection to the Father active, deep and consistent. Look at these examples:

"Now in the morning, having risen a long while before daylight, He went out and departed to a solitary place; and there He prayed." Mark 1:35

"So He Himself often withdrew into the wilderness and prayed." Luke 5:16

"Now it came to pass in those days that He went out to the mountain to pray, and continued all night in prayer to God." Luke 6:12

God cannot be shocked by anything we say in prayer. As a result, honest prayer is a freeing experience. In the Bible, psalmists accuse, question and scold God. They also celebrate, confess and exalt.

Richard J. Foster, author of *Prayer*, admits, "Who we are — not who we want to be — is the only offering we have to give."

"Let us therefore come boldly to the throne of grace, that we may obtain mercy and find grace to help in time of need." Hebrews 4:16

Some have found the acronym ACTS to be helpful in praying.

A = **Adoration** — praising/admiring God for who He is

C = **Confession** — we acknowledge our sins and seek forgiveness

T = **Thanks** — for all He has done for us and for others

S = **Supplication** — we submit our requests for ourselves and others. Remember to ask, "What would You have me do?"

IN YOUR OWN WORDS

WHAT CAN YOU DO TO MAKE PRAYER A GREATER PART OF YOUR LIFE?

....

....

....

....

....

"The most important thing that ever happens in prayer," reflects Brennan Manning, "is letting ourselves be loved by God. 'Be still and know that I am God' (Psalm 46). It's like slipping into a tub of hot water and letting God's love wash over us, enfold us…. The awareness of being loved brings a touch of lightness and a tint of brightness and sometimes, for no apparent reason, a smile plays at the corner of your mouth."

A true friend is one who knows the song of your heart and can sing it back to you when you forget the words.

Author unknown

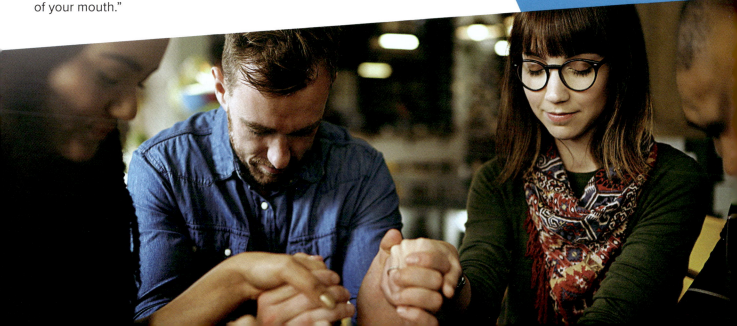

FOUR WAYS TO DEVELOP TRUST

1. BIBLE STUDY

The Bible helps us to grow in every area of life. We can turn to the Bible to give wisdom, encouragement and ideas of what to do. Start by reading any one of the gospels (Matthew, Mark, Luke or John) and let God speak to you through His Word.

"Your word is a lamp to my feet." Psalm 119:105

2. WORSHIP

Corporate

As we follow Jesus, we learn to appreciate and love His church as a diverse, humble community of believers. A healthy congregation does more than just show up for a sermon. They share one another's burdens and unite to accomplish what is impossible to do alone.

"And let us consider one another in order to stir up love and good works, not forsaking the assembling of ourselves together, as is the manner of some, but exhorting one another, and so much the more as you see the day approaching." Hebrews 10:24, 25

Music is a language that touches our emotions. Songs can be used as weapons against discouragement. A simple act such as singing in a choir has even been found to increase function of the immune system.

"I will bless the Lord at all times; His praise shall continually be in my mouth. My soul makes its boast in the Lord; let the humble hear and be glad." Psalm 34:1, 2

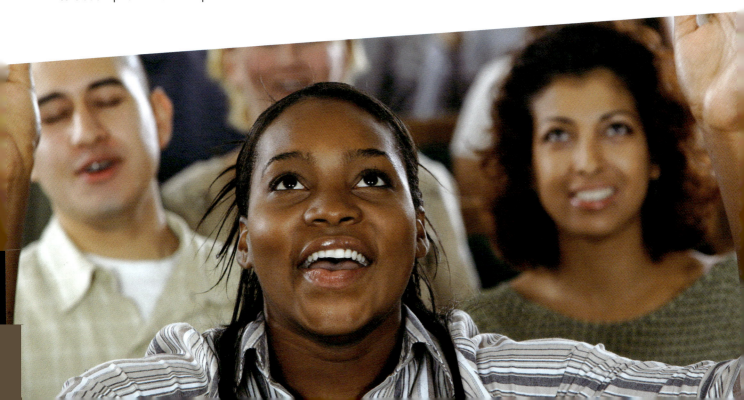

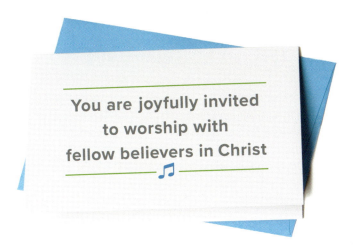

You are joyfully invited
to worship with
fellow believers in Christ
♫

Individual

We live busy lives. Jesus warned that "the cares of this world" can choke out trust in God (Matthew 13:22). Those who set aside time in the morning for worship and commitment find their life brightened with hope. Just praying, "God, please order my day," brings surprising effectiveness.

"My voice You shall hear in the morning, O Lord;
In the morning I will direct it to You, and I will look up."
Psalm 5:3

There will be times when no other help is available and we need to trust God alone. As the saying goes, "God has no grandchildren." *You* are God's child.

3. FASTING

"'When you fast, do not be like the hypocrites, with a sad countenance. For they disfigure their faces that they may appear to men to be fasting. Assuredly, I say to you, they have their reward. But you, when you fast, anoint your head and wash your face, so that you do not appear to men to be fasting, but to your Father who is in the secret place; and your Father who sees in secret will reward you openly.'" Matthew 6:16-18

Fasting is a way of restricting food to a level that would not normally be consumed. Restricting food has been found to increase immune function, weight loss, decrease the rate of aging and increase the average and maximum lifespan. Food restriction reduces cancer formation, kidney disease and in experimental models of Alzheimer's and Parkinson's diseases, it increases resistance of neurons to dysfunction and degeneration. Fasting gives our body a focused, healthy break.

Some people aren't able to totally fast from food. Sometimes they follow a simpler diet or leave off desserts. Others find that a fast from television or the Internet for a span of time helps to clear the mind for God.

4. SERVING OTHERS

Another type of fast is to turn away from the abundance of envy, blame and self-centeredness that surrounds us and serve others. Trust grows as we ourselves become more involved in God's restoration project in this world. God's "chosen fast" is described in Isaiah's marvelous chapter 58.

"Is this not the fast that I have chosen: to loose bonds of wickedness, to undo the heavy burdens, to let the oppressed go free, and that You break every yoke? Is it not to share Your bread with the hungry, and that You bring to Your house the poor who are cast out; when You see the naked, that You cover him, and not hide Yourself from Your own flesh? Then Your light shall break forth like the morning, Your healing shall spring forth speedily." Isaiah 58:6-8

Killing Jesus was like trying to destroy a dandelion seed-head by blowing on it.

Walter Wink

TRUST IN THE BLESSED HOPE

What is the aim, the grand design of all our trust? What keeps us going even in the midst of difficult struggles? As Titus 2:13 describes, we are "looking for the blessed hope and glorious appearing of our great God and Savior Jesus Christ." Believers in Christ long for the day when He will return and finally set all creation free. But how can we trust that this wonderful time will truly take place? By trusting His promises:

"I am the resurrection and the life. Those who believe in Me, even though they die, will live." John 11:25

"In My Father's house are many mansions; if it were not so, I would have told you. I go to prepare a place for you. And if I go to prepare a place for you, I will come again and receive you to Myself: that where I am, there you will be also." John 14:2, 3

Notice what Jesus says: "I would have told you if it weren't the case." Yes, He will come back for us.

"So Christ, having been offered once to bear the sins of many, will appear a second time, not to deal with sin, but to save those who are eagerly waiting for him." Hebrews 9:28

Jesus' Second Coming is not for Him to deal with sin (He dealt with sin already on the cross), but to rescue those who are yearning to see Him. Those who place their trust in Him not only live better lives now, but will finally receive their reward. The Bible describes the Second Coming as seen by His followers.

"And it will be said in that day: 'Behold, this is our God; we have waited for Him, and He will save us. This is the Lord; we have waited for Him; we will be glad and rejoice in His salvation.'" Isaiah 25:9

Life's true conclusion has not yet appeared, yet we know that it will.

In November of 1996, a cyclone ravished the coast of India near Masalidippa, flooding villages and killing more than 1,000 people. In addition, 1,300 fishermen were reported missing in their boats. The grieving families looked out to sea for their fathers, brothers and husbands, but what hope did they have? A day passed. Two days. Three days. Four days. The nation gave up the fishermen for dead.

On the fifth day, people on the beach spotted something on the horizon. A flotilla of 162 boats sailed home to a joyous, unbelievable welcome.

This is only a small picture of what will take place at Christ's return. Don't ever give up hope. Keep trusting in Him.

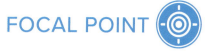

FOCAL POINT

WHICH TRUST PATHWAY WILL YOU PURSUE THIS WEEK? WHAT DO YOU WANT THE RESULTS TO BE?

....

....

....

....

....

....

....

....

....

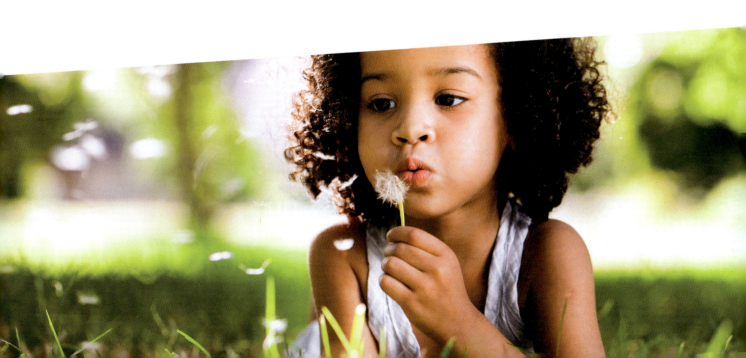

LIFE APPLICATION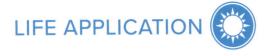

Take a moment to reflect on this CREATION Life study on trust in God.

WHAT PRINCIPLES HAVE YOU LEARNED THAT YOU WANT TO APPLY IN YOUR LIFE?

....

....

....

....

NOW, CREATE A PERSONAL GOAL TO STRENGTHEN YOUR TRUST IN GOD.

....

....

....

....

Examples of goals for trust in God:

My goal is to spend 20 minutes each morning in personal devotion and prayer.

My goal is to say at least three times each day, "God, what would You have me do?" (And then be quiet, listening for a godly impression).

My goal is to fast once a month with a fast of my choice.

My goal is to join a loving church community this week.

My goal is to give my worries and fears to God every time they try to take over.

"You will keep Him in perfect peace whose mind is stayed on You, because he trusts in You." Isaiah 26:3

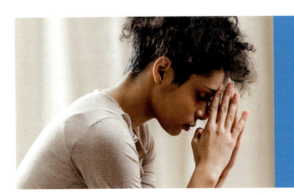

I have been driven many times to my knees by the overwhelming conviction that I had nowhere else to go. Abraham Lincoln

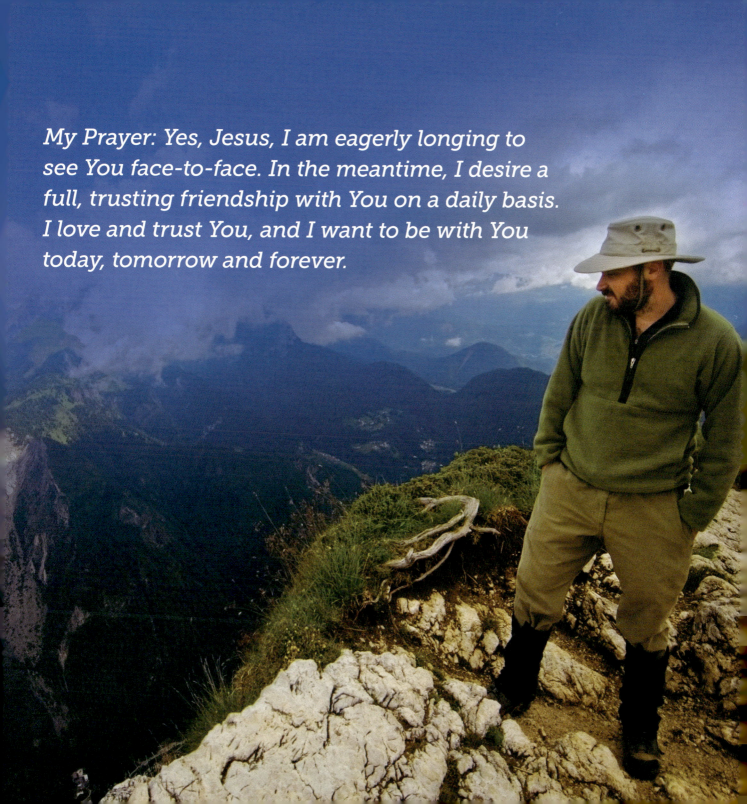

My Prayer: Yes, Jesus, I am eagerly longing to see You face-to-face. In the meantime, I desire a full, trusting friendship with You on a daily basis. I love and trust You, and I want to be with You today, tomorrow and forever.

SMALL GROUP DISCUSSION QUESTIONS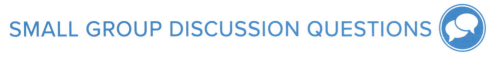

1. **WHICH BIBLE TEXT ON TRUST IMPACTED YOU MOST?**

    ....

    ....

    ....

2. **DO YOU THINK IT'S POSSIBLE TO TRUST AS MUCH AS CANON GOLDSMITH? WOULDN'T WE GET "BURNED" OFTEN?**

    ....

    ....

    ....

3. **WHY IS PRAYER SO DIFFICULT? WHAT HAVE YOU PERSONALLY FOUND THAT HELPS?**

    ....

    ....

    ....

4. **"LOVING GOD REQUIRES OBEDIENCE." DO YOU AGREE? WHAT HAPPENS WHEN WE FAIL TO OBEY?**

    ....

    ....

    ....

5. **HOW DO YOU GET OVER PROBLEMS WITH FINDING TIME FOR INDIVIDUAL WORSHIP? FOR THOSE WHO HAVE FOUND SOLUTIONS, DID YOU EVER STRUGGLE AND NEARLY GIVE UP?**

....

....

....

....

6. **WHY DO YOU THINK PEOPLE ARE AFRAID OF THE SECOND COMING? WHAT WOULD HELP THEM OVERCOME THEIR FEAR?**

....

....

....

....

7. **SHARE ONE OF YOUR TRUST GOALS WITH THE GROUP. HOW COULD THE GROUP HELP YOU REACH THIS GOAL?**

....

....

....

....

....

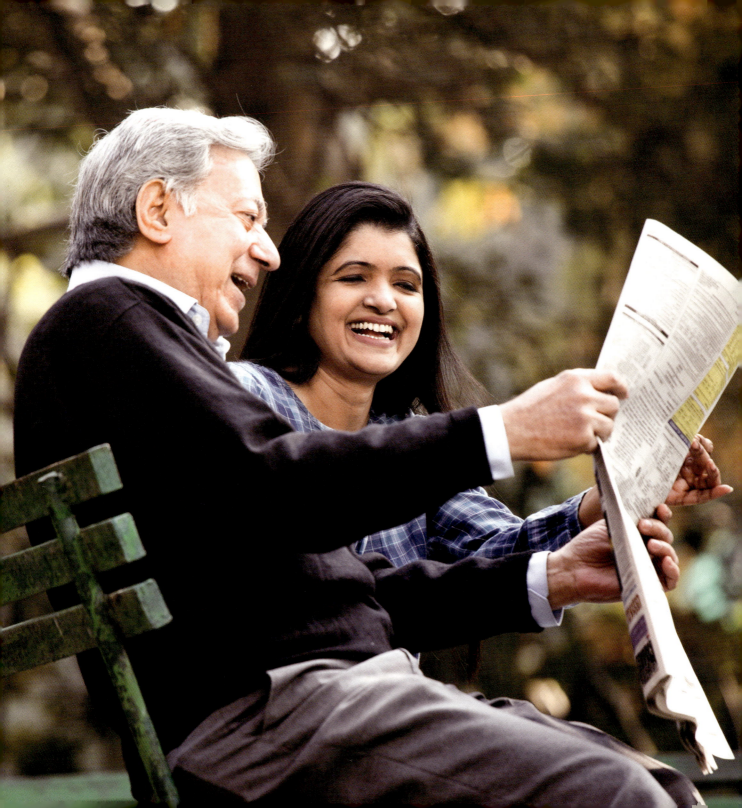

INTERPERSONAL
RELATIONSHIPS

I give you a new commandment, that you love one another. Just as I have loved you, you should love one another. John 13:34

Do relationships impact our well-being? Think about it: Do we value kind words spoken from a close friend or a warm hug at a difficult time? Yet we have to admit that these same relationships also bring some of life's biggest challenges.

That's where God comes in. God supplies us with interpersonal tools of tact, truth and time. In addition, we remember the first lesson of CREATION Life — choice. We always have a choice in how we will respond to and treat others.

Sidney Harris, writing in the *Chicago Daily News*, described walking to the newsstand with a friend. His friend bought a paper and thanked the newsboy politely. The young man replied merely with a grunt.

"A solemn fellow, isn't he?" Harris commented afterward.

"Yes, he's that way every day."

"Yet I noticed that you went out of your way to be courteous to him."

The friend replied, *"Why should I let him decide how I am going to act?"*

You can approach your relationships as a victim or as an agent of grace and change. The bottom line is this: You decide.

Where I Am *(Place a mark on the line to show what you're feeling right now.)*

I'm basically unsatisfied with my relationships.

My interpersonal relationships bring peace and joy.

Dr. Dean Ornish was one of the first to scientifically document the reversibility of heart disease through diet and exercise. However, in his book *Love and Survival: The Scientific Basis for the Healing Power of Intimacy*, he explains the even more profound impact love and intimacy have on our health:

> I'm not aware of any other factor in medicine — not diet, not smoking, not exercise, not stress, not genetics, not drugs, not surgery — that has a greater impact on our quality of life, incidence of illness and the premature death from all causes.

In Guatemala City, a study was conducted on two groups of pregnant women. One group went through labor alone, while another group had constant support from a friendly companion known as a doula, or labor coach. The doula accompanied each mom-to-be from the moment they were admitted to the final moments of delivery. "The duration of labor in the group of women left alone was 19.3 hours, compared to only 8.7 hours for the women with the doula."[1]

The vital importance of intimacy and healthy touch was also highlighted by the case of two newborn twins, Kyrie and Brielle, who changed the care of premature babies in hospitals all over the world.

Kyrie and Brielle were born 12 weeks early. Immediately the doctors knew something was wrong. While Kyrie was sleeping and gaining weight, Brielle was not faring well. She had breathing and heart rate troubles resulting in low oxygen levels in her blood. When Brielle was at her worst, a nurse decided to try something she had recently heard about at a seminar. It was a simple procedure, but strictly forbidden by hospital policy.

With the parents' permission, the nurse took Brielle out of the incubator and placed her with her sister Kyrie. The two girls hadn't seen each other since birth. Immediately, Brielle calmed down and began to sleep better. Her blood oxygen levels improved and she gained weight. Occasionally, Kyrie would put her arm around her sister while they slept. Brielle eventually made a full recovery.

"Two are better than one, because they have a good reward for their toil. For if they fall, one will lift up the other; but woe to one who is alone and falls and does not have another to help." Ecclesiastes 4:9, 10

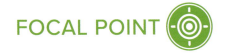

FOCAL POINT

IF I HAD TO COUNT ON ONE PERSON IN THIS WORLD, IT WOULD BE

....

UNITY IN DIVERSITY

In His longest-recorded prayer, Jesus prayed for His followers:

"That they may all be one, as You, Father, are in Me, and I in You; that they also may be one in Us, that the world may believe that You sent Me." John 17:21

Maybe you think being in unity with God and with one another means you must first lose your individuality. But know, the God who makes billions of variations on snowflakes and leaves, dimples on knees and scents on the breeze, intentionally makes people different. As Christians and children of God, we can learn to *appreciate* and *celebrate* our individual differences.

"There are diversities of gifts, but the same Spirit. There are differences of ministries, but the same Lord. And there are diversities of activities, but it is the same God who works all in all." 1 Corinthians 12:4-6

Staying true to ourselves isn't easy. The poet E. E. Cummings observed, "To be nobody-but-yourself — in a world which is doing its best, night and day, to make you everybody else — means to fight the hardest battle which any human being can fight, and never stop fighting." Remember that God created you as a unique, cherished and priceless person.

IN YOUR OWN WORDS

DESCRIBE YOURSELF WHEN YOU ARE AUTHENTICALLY YOU.

....

....

....

....

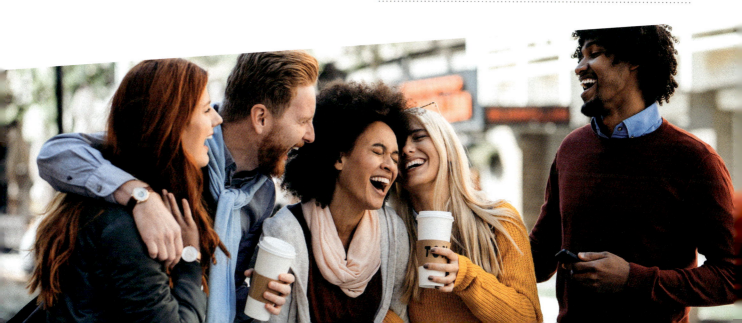

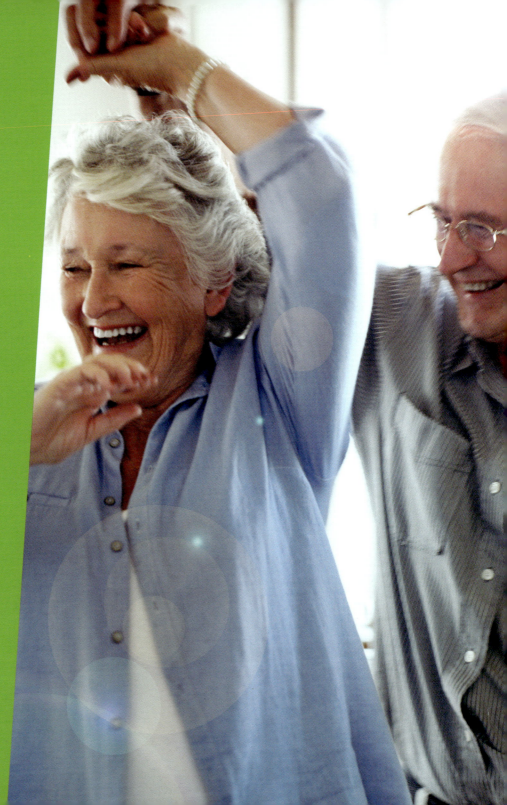

Be loving, responsible, fun, strong, gentle and loyal.

ALL IN THE FAMILY

Oftentimes, the people we find the most difficult to *get along with* are those who we are closest to — our families. Our feelings for each other run so deep, and our shared history is so long and complicated that opportunities for conflict are always present. How can we minimize these conflicts?

Jesus provided a superb example of taking care of family. Even on the cross, He took time to acknowledge the importance of His mother and asked His friend John to look after her.

"When Jesus therefore saw His mother, and the disciple whom He loved standing by, He said to His mother, 'Woman, behold your son!' Then He said to the disciple, 'Behold your mother!' And from that hour that disciple took her to his own home." John 19:26, 27

Consider the Bible's counsel for family relationships. For those who are not married, God has promised to be there for us.

"For your Maker is your husband, the Lord of hosts is His name; and your redeemer is the Holy One of Israel; He is called the God of the whole earth." Isaiah 54:5

The Bible also has advice about how husbands and wives should interact with each other within marriage.

"Live joyfully with the wife [husband] whom you love all the days of your vain life which He has given you under the sun." Ecclesiastes 9:9

In other words, choose to be happily content with the woman or man you married. In addition, you can be the person your partner longs for — loving, responsible, fun, strong, gentle and loyal.

Our society is suffering from a disintegration of marriages. Affairs destroy the lives of too many couples. How can we affair-proof our marriages? By carrying God's love and warnings within our hearts.

"For the commandment is a lamp and the teaching a light, and the reproofs of discipline are the way of life, to preserve you from the evil woman [or man], from the smooth tongue of the adventuress. Do not desire her beauty in your heart, and do not let her capture you with her eyelashes. For a harlot may be hired for a crust of bread, but an adulteress stalks a man's very life.... He who commits adultery has no sense; he who does it destroys himself. Wounds and dishonor will he get, and his disgrace will not be wiped away." Proverbs 6:23-26, 32, 33

When a couple follows God's commands, it protects them from the misery adultery brings. In fact, that's the whole point of God's commandments: to stop suffering, increase freedom, nurture peace and deliver joy.

A massive study of 90,000 teenagers across the United States collected data to determine the factors most likely to protect them from harm and help them enjoy an abundant life. The one word that summarized the research above all the others was *connectedness*. Teens who felt connected to family, church, school and their community were far less likely to participate in behaviors that put them at risk.[2]

"She opens her mouth with wisdom, and on her tongue is the law of kindness." Proverbs 31:26

"Fathers, do not provoke your children, lest they become discouraged." **Colossians 3:21**

J. Allan Peterson writes about "teaching a lesson" to children.

> I read about a small boy who was consistently late coming home from school. His parents warned him one day that he must be home on time that afternoon, but nevertheless he arrived later than ever. His mother met him at the door and said nothing. His father met him in the living room and said nothing.
>
> At dinner that night, the boy looked at his plate. There was a slice of bread and a glass of water. He looked at his father's full plate and then at his father, but his father remained silent. The boy was crushed.
>
> The father waited for the full impact to sink in, then quietly took the boy's plate and placed it in front of himself. He took his own plate of meat and potatoes, put it in front of the boy and smiled at his son.
>
> When the boy grew to be a man, he said, "All my life I've known what God is like by what my father did that night."

The Bible counsels us not to "provoke" our children. When someone we love and admire treats us harshly or berates us verbally it leaves lasting scars of discouragement. But when parents always respect their children and *each other,* this multiplies the security and health of the entire family.

LIFE APPLICATION

WHAT PRACTICAL STEPS CAN I TAKE TO MAKE A DIFFERENCE IN MY FAMILY?

....

....

....

....

....

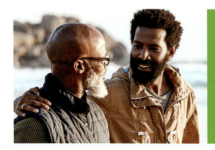

You can easily judge the character of a man by how he treats those who can do nothing for him. *James D. Mills*

HOW SHOULD I ACT TOWARD MY ENEMIES?

In life, we all encounter people who are hard to get along with. Sometimes these relationships can become bitter and even hostile, but the Bible makes it clear: these people are not our true enemies.

"We do not wrestle against flesh and blood, but against principalities, against powers, against the rulers of the darkness of this age, against spiritual hosts of wickedness in the heavenly places." Ephesians 6:12

It's helpful to recognize we all share a common tendency to distrust and judge those who are not like us. Oddly, the less we relate to people the more certain we seem to be of their motives. But God gives us another idea that causes a radical shift in our thinking.

"You have heard that it was said, 'You shall love your neighbor and hate your enemy.' But I say to you, love your enemies and pray for those who persecute you, so that you may be [children] of your Father who is in heaven; for He makes His sun rise on the evil and on the good, and sends rain on the just and on the unjust.'" Matthew 5:43-45

"'If your enemy is hungry, feed him; if he is thirsty, give him a drink; for in so doing you will heap coals of fire on his head.' Do not be overcome by evil, but overcome evil with good." Romans 12:20, 21

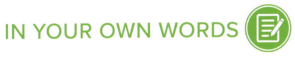

IN YOUR OWN WORDS

WHAT DO THESE VERSES TELL US ABOUT HOW WE ARE TO TREAT "ENEMIES"?

....

....

....

....

....

....

GRACIOUS LIVING

Grace is unmerited favor delivered through *forgiveness, acceptance* and *sharing*. As we receive God's grace, He asks that we extend it to others. Yet grace is far easier to talk about than to live out. For example, consider the first component of grace: forgiveness. Why should we forgive others when they have seriously hurt us?

"If you forgive others the wrongs they have done, your heavenly Father will also forgive you; but if you do not forgive others, then the wrongs you have done will not be forgiven by your Father." Matthew 6, 14, 15

We must forgive to be forgiven ourselves. The command to forgive is as essential to our health as is the quality of our rest, exercise and nutrition. Think about how our physical bodies function. When we incur an injury, the safest remedy is to clean the wound to prevent infection. If the wound becomes infected it must be treated, and the longer the wound is left untreated the more the infection spreads until the results are fatal.

When we're wounded emotionally, we must also clean the wound, and the only way to do that is to forgive. Otherwise, the wound will expand, infecting other areas of our lives. We probably won't feel like forgiving at all. It might be the most difficult thing we've ever done, but followers of Jesus respond regardless of their feelings.

What do we mean when we say "forgive"? It may be helpful to note first what forgiving is not. Forgiving is not avoiding dealing with an incident. That brand of indifference creates greater conflict down the road.

Forgiving is also not agreeing with the wrong that was done. Some people might think saying, "I forgive you" really means, "What you have done *isn't* wrong." But that's not the case at all. We don't have to worry that forgiving someone for anything will mean we agree with what was done.

Forgiving simply means letting go of the wrong that was done to us. We give it to God, we no longer hold it against the person, and we move on in our relationship. In the process, we free ourselves from the slavery of bitterness and resentment, no matter how much we have been hurt.

"And when they had come to the place called Calvary, there they crucified Him, and the criminals, one on the right hand and the other on the left. Then Jesus said, 'Father, forgive them, for they do not know what they do.'" Luke 23:33, 34

When we refuse to forgive, we do terrible damage to ourselves. An unforgiving attitude limits our creativity, constricts our sense of humor and saps our enjoyment of life. Perhaps most tragically, refusing to forgive reduces our ability to love others — even those whom we don't need to forgive.

We say it's hard to forgive, but forgiving makes life easier, not harder. Corrie Ten Boom, who survived a Nazi concentration camp, points out the physical consequences of not forgiving.

I knew (forgiving) not only as a commandment of God, but as a daily experience. Since the end of the war I had had a home in Holland for victims of Nazi brutality. Those who were able to forgive their former enemies were able also to return to the outside world and rebuild their lives, no matter what the physical scars. Those who nursed their bitterness remained invalids. It was as simple and as horrible as that.

One notable example of forgiveness was demonstrated by Clara Barton, founder of the American Red Cross. A friend of Barton's once reminded her of something especially cruel that someone had done to her years before, but Clara didn't seem to recall the incident. "Don't you remember it?" her friend asked.

"No," came the reply, "I distinctly remember forgetting it."

"Therefore, as the elect of God, holy and beloved, put on tender mercies, kindness, humility, meekness, longsuffering; bearing with one another, and forgiving one another, if anyone has a complaint against another; even as Christ forgave you, so you also must do." Colossians 3:12, 13

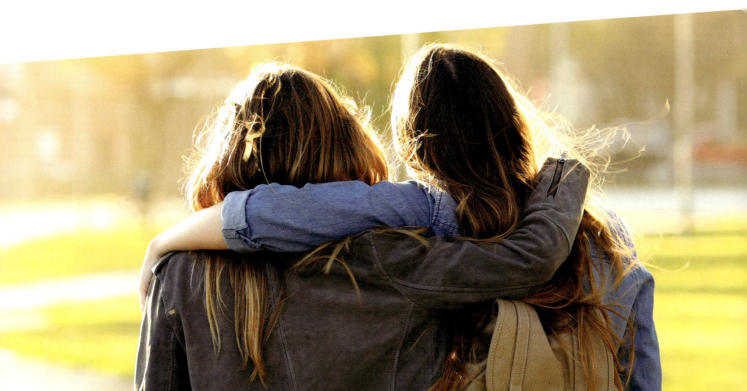

But what happens when we're wounded afresh, when feelings of outrage and pain arise even more intensely than before? Do we have to forgive again?

Sometimes the pain may be retrieved from the subconscience. Impressions stored in our long-term memory can be recalled years later. A name, a room or a smell may trigger the memory of that horrible experience you thought you had put behind you. You may wonder, *Maybe I never really forgave the first time*. But don't be discouraged. Experiencing the feelings again doesn't mean you never forgave the first time. And feelings in themselves aren't ever wrong — it's what we choose to do with those feelings that makes the difference.

When hurtful memories appear and the issue is re-opened, there is only one way to keep the door closed. We must forgive again. It is the only way we can put the past behind us and start anew.

"Then Peter came to Him and said, 'Lord, how often shall my brother sin against me, and I forgive him? Up to seven times?' Jesus said to him, 'I do not say to you, up to seven times, but up to seventy times seven.'" Matthew 18:21, 22

FOCAL POINT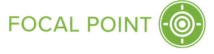

On the line below, write the initials of people you need to forgive. Set yourself free by asking God to help you forgive them. Give the incident and person to God, and move on with your life. Pray. Do it now.

....

....

....

ACCEPTING OTHERS

"Now all the tax collectors and sinners were coming near to listen to Him. And the Pharisees and the scribes were grumbling and saying, 'This fellow welcomes sinners and eats with them.'"   Luke 15:1, 2

Acceptance is *affirming the infinite worth of another person*, no matter what he or she has done. In this context, accepting doesn't mean we agree with a person's poor choices or endorse their ideas, but it does mean we respect the dignity and value of another human being.

A favorite tactic of schoolteachers is to make two boys who have been fighting work on a job — just the two of them. What often happens as a result? The fighters become friends. By working closely together they begin to see a new side to the other person. They learn to settle their differences and work together in peace.

"Judge not, that you be not judged."   Matthew 7:1

Nothing devastates love more than a critical spirit. In fact, Jesus directed His most scathing attacks at the critics. Jesus came to build His kingdom on the foundation of strong, loving relationships. He knew a critical attitude would damage relationships and ultimately destroy them. That's why we are told not to judge but to discern: "Those who are spiritual discern all things" (1 Corinthians 2:15, NRSV).

You may be wondering, "What's the difference?" Think of it this way: Judging evaluates the actor; discerning evaluates the action.

All of us carry incomplete knowledge about others. This realization should fill us with humility and compassion in all of our interactions.

"Live in harmony with one another; do not be haughty, but associate with the lowly; do not claim to be wiser than you are."   Romans 12:16

> *Not forgiving someone is like drinking rat poison and waiting for the rat to die.*
>
> Anne Lamott

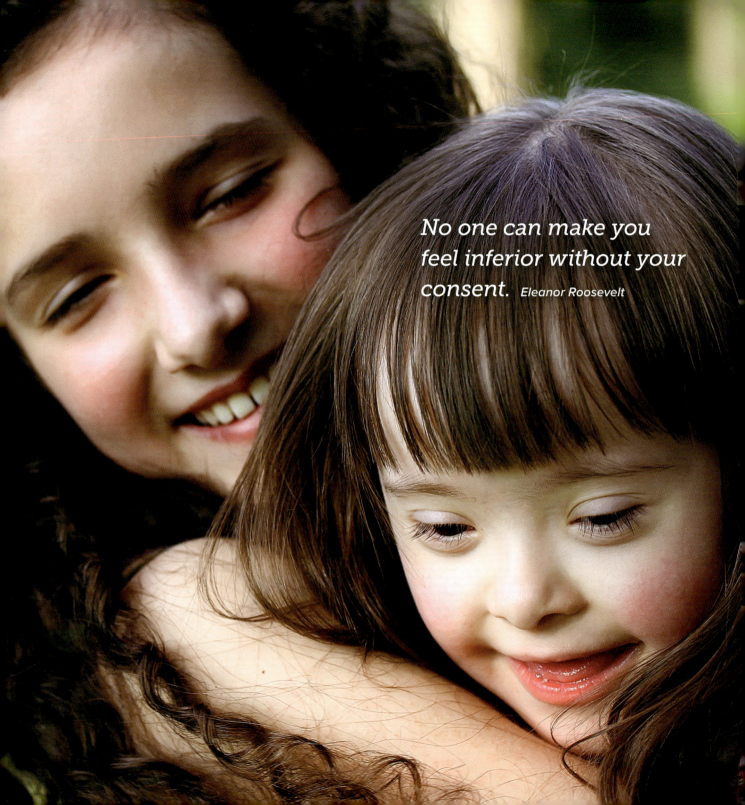

No one can make you feel inferior without your consent. *Eleanor Roosevelt*

IN YOUR OWN WORDS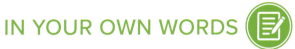

WHAT HELPS ME MOST TO ACCEPT THOSE WHO ARE DIFFERENT FROM ME IS:

....

....

....

....

Jesus was often seen in the company of people who were well-known sinners. He even seemed at ease with these people (which is one of the reasons the religious leaders were so critical of Him). These sinners were also comfortable with Jesus.

Jesus could accept sinners because He saw them for what they really were — people with needs and weaknesses. But along with these He also saw their burning desire for something better in life. God wants to open our vision, to see others' possibilities, their loneliness and their longings.

"The one who comes to Me I will by no means cast out." John 6:37

"God demonstrates His own love toward us, in that while we were still sinners, Christ died for us." Romans 5:8

Because we know we're loved and accepted, we become changed. An apple tree doesn't bear fruit to become an apple tree. An apple tree bears fruit *because* it is an apple tree.

I BELIEVE I AM LOVED AND ACCEPTED BY GOD, JUST AS I AM. ☐ YES ☐ NO

I SEEM TO HAVE THE MOST TROUBLE ACCEPTING PEOPLE WHO ARE:

☐ STUBBORN ☐ SELFISH ☐ JEALOUS

☐ UNKIND ☐ FILTHY ☐ LAZY

☐ ARROGANT ☐ GOSSIPY ☐ HOSTILE

☐ DISRESPECTFUL ☐ —————————

I BELIEVE JESUS ACCEPTS THESE PEOPLE JUST AS THEY ARE. ☐ YES ☐ NO

RIGHT NOW I HAVE TROUBLE ACCEPTING THESE PEOPLE: (WRITE THEIR INITIALS)

....

Accepting decision: I admit I have had difficulty accepting people with these characteristics. I realize, however, that I am accepted by my God, and that because of God's acceptance I can accept these people. This does not obligate me to approve of their behavior. This simply means I will always love them, I will always openly accept them in the name of Jesus Christ.

(Signed) _____

"Create in me a clean heart, O God, and renew a steadfast spirit within me." Psalm 51:10

SHARING AND CARING

"And do not forget to do good and to share with others, for with such sacrifices God is well pleased." Hebrews 13:16

A survey by the Institute for the Advancement of Health was conducted of people who volunteered throughout the United States from large cities to rural areas. The study found 95 percent of those who had regular personal contact with the individuals they helped were blessed with a feel-good sensation that became known as "helper's high." However, if the contact was not both regular and personal, the feeling vanished.

One volunteer wrote, "Some months ago I was so stressed out that I could barely get four hours sleep at night and I had all sorts of aches and pains. I had even tried antidepressant and anti-anxiety drugs, but to no avail. Then I found out firsthand that it is love that truly heals. When I do nice things, I definitely feel a physical response. For me it is mostly a relaxation of muscles that I hadn't even realized had been tensed.... I can now sleep well at night, and most of my aches and pains have disappeared."[3]

In practical terms, helping others produces long-term health benefits, including relief from back pain and headaches, lowered blood pressure and a reduction of overeating and alcohol and drug abuse.

Defending the dignity of those we help always brings the best results. In a famous statement, Lila Watson, an Australian Aboriginal woman, responded to mission workers, "If you have come to help me, you are wasting your time. But if you have come because your liberation is bound up with mine, then let us walk together."

"The generous soul will be made rich, and he who waters will also be watered himself." Proverbs 11:25

The true follower of Jesus doesn't participate in blaming and complaining. Instead, she fixes relationships through creative, redemptive action. Viktor Frankl proclaims, "Freedom is only part of the story and half the truth.... That is why I recommend that the Statue of Liberty on the East Coast be supplemented by the Statue of Responsibility on the West Coast."

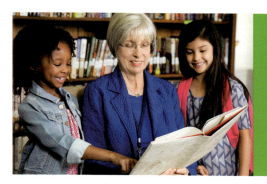

It is hard for a free fish to understand what is happening to a hooked one. Karl A. Menninger

LIFE APPLICATION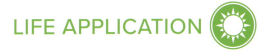

What can you do to minister to others? Keep these principles in mind:

- Have personal contact with the person you help.

- Ensure frequent helping, with a rough goal of two hours a week.

- Do a task that you are already equipped to do or will be trained to do.

- Pursue an opportunity that is connected to your personal interests. Some ideas might include volunteering at an animal shelter or tutoring in a public school. Perhaps you could be a "big brother or sister," take meals to shut-ins or share songs at an assisted living facility. The possibilities are endless.

WHAT SHARING IDEA APPEALS TO YOU?
WHO COULD YOU DO THIS WITH?

....

....

....

....

....

....

....

....

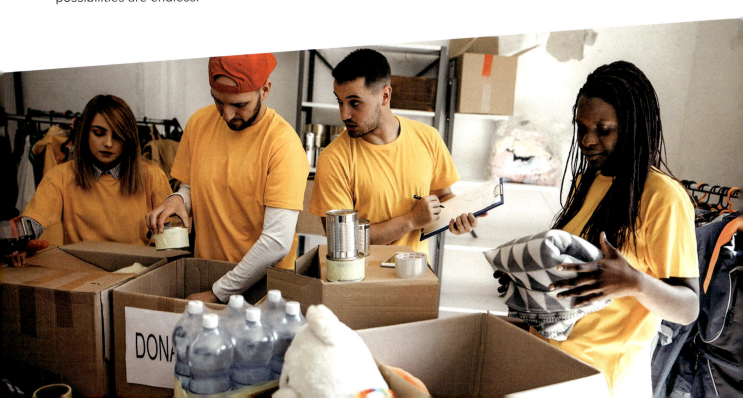

COMMUNICATION: THE KEY TO LIFE

In his book *Why Am I Afraid to Tell You Who I Am?* John Powell shows that communication involves five deepening levels:

LEVEL 5 — CLICHÉ CONVERSATION

The most superficial level, this type of talk is quick and safe. These are the "Good morning," "How are you?" "I'm fine" comments we say in passing. While this communication is necessary in our society, we must seek to move deeper.

LEVEL 4 — REPORTING THE FACTS

At this level, we report news happenings or may even share small stories, but we don't commit ourselves to commenting on how these events and actions make us feel.

LEVEL 3 — IDEAS AND JUDGMENTS

Friendly conversation begins as we share our thoughts and ideas on different subjects. Because this level involves a personal element it also carries some risk. Some people have difficulty functioning at this level and retreat to previous levels.

LEVEL 2 — FEELINGS AND EMOTIONS

Here we begin to share our feelings about facts, ideas and judgments. When these emotions are revealed, a tender part of ourselves is exposed. This level is vital to meaningful communication.

LEVEL 1 — OPEN AND TRUTHFUL COMMUNICATION

Communication on this level is reserved for only a few close people in our lives. It is here we are the most vulnerable. But that's what true love is all about. *We can never be totally accepted until we provide the opportunity for someone to know who we truly are.* This requires us to be completely open and truthful.

Many people live their entire lives without ever reaching level one communication with anyone. Some people never allow themselves to communicate on level two. But these people are missing out. They're missing the joy and excitement of living a confident, candid, caring life.

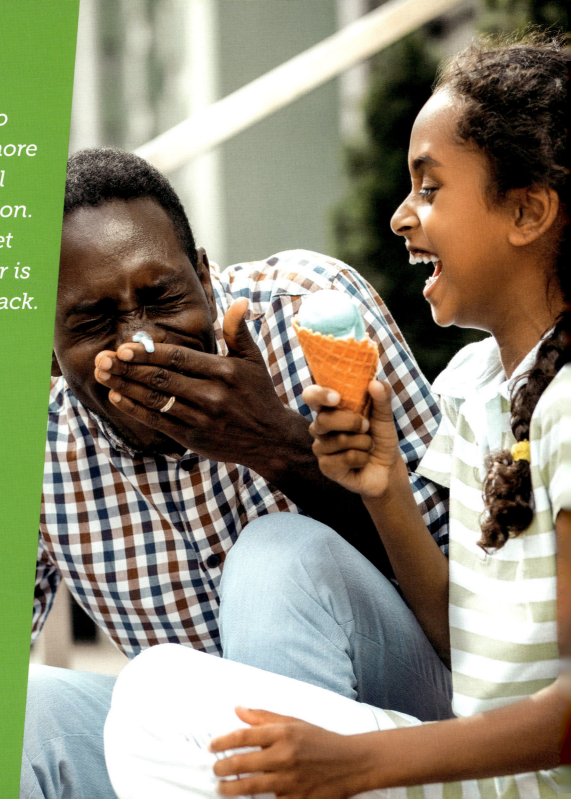

My Prayer:
God, I want to
experience more
open, truthful
communication.
Help me to get
over whatever is
holding me back.
Thank You.

USING "I LANGUAGE"

"There is one who speaks like the piercings of a sword, but the tongue of the wise promotes health." Proverbs 12:18

"Your jokes are dumb."

"You're always so negative."

"You never mind your own business!"

These are examples of "you language." Words like "you," "always," and "never" can be toxic to a discussion and arouse defensiveness in the listener. Think about how you feel when these kinds of comments are directed at you.

Fortunately, there is a better way for us to communicate with each other. "I language" portrays behavior without making accusatory remarks. A complete "I" statement describes

- the other person's *behavior*,

- your *feelings* and

- the *consequences* the other's behavior has for you.

Pleasant words are like a honeycomb, sweetness to the soul and health to the bones. Proverbs 16:24

"Mentioning my mistakes in front of other people (Behavior) makes me feel embarrassed [Feeling]. I'm afraid they'll think I'm stupid [Consequence]."

"Because there was no one to pick me up on time [Behavior] I was late for the conference [Consequence]. It made me feel that my job and priorities aren't important [Feeling]."

Can you see how this is a better approach? It's difficult to argue with "I statements." They enable people to truly listen. As Mortimer Adler suggests, "Don't say 'Look' when you mean 'Please listen.'"

LIFE APPLICATION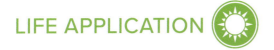

Develop your skill using "I language." (Make this your life practice).

CREATE BEHAVIOR/FEELING/CONSEQUENCE ALTERNATIVES FOR THESE STATEMENTS

"WOULD YOU QUIT CRITICIZING ME?"

....

....

"YOU ALWAYS THINK YOU'RE RIGHT!"

....

....

In *Notes to Myself*, Hugh Prather observes, "Our marriage used to suffer from arguments that were too short. Now we argue long enough to find out what the argument is about."

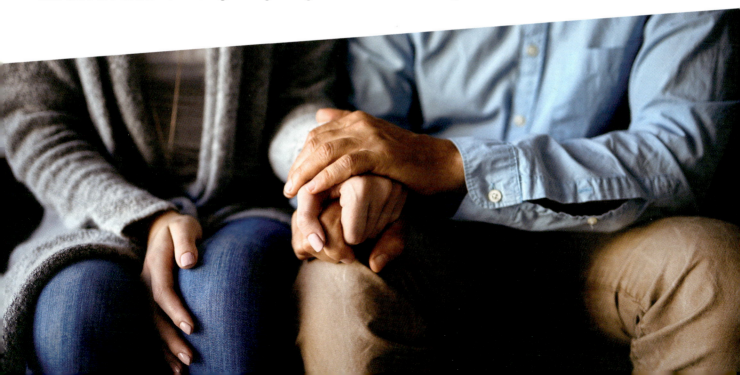

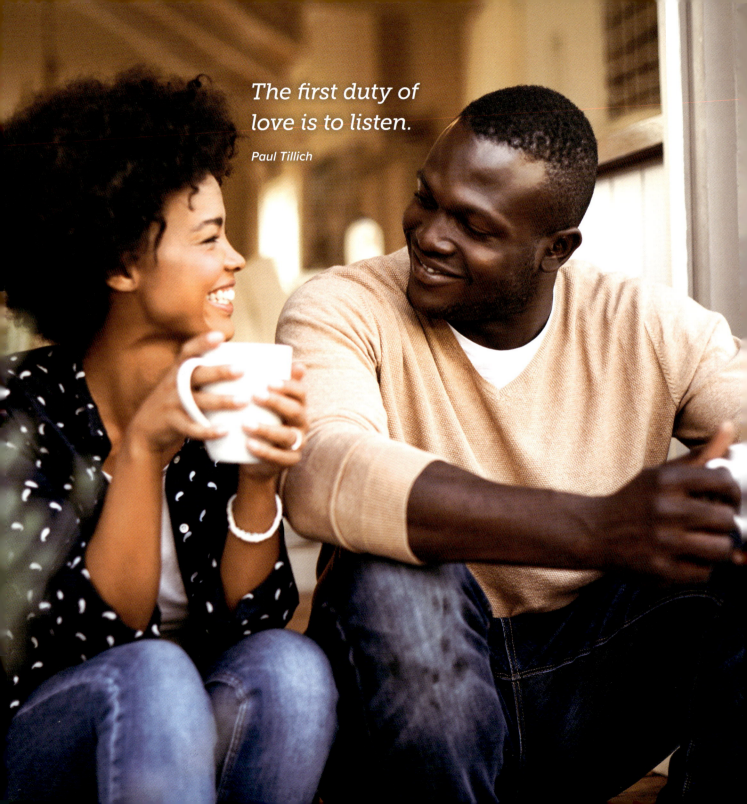

The first duty of
love is to listen.

Paul Tillich

LANGUAGE MATTERS

In her book *I Only Say This Because I Love You,* Deborah Tannen maintains that all conversation hinges on control or connection. As you converse with anyone, ask yourself, *Am I seeking to control or to connect with this person?*

Take a healthy approach to conversation. First, carefully listen for the prompting of the Holy Spirit before saying words that imply control.

"When the Spirit of truth comes, He will guide you into all the truth." John 16:13

Learn to cultivate self-control as a mindful discipline. This will help you to avoid the realm of gossip.

"A gossip goes about telling secrets, but one who is trustworthy in spirit keeps a confidence."
Proverbs 11:13

"Even fools who keep silent are considered wise; when they close their lips, they are deemed intelligent."
Proverbs 17:28

Finally, embrace the truth, but always share it with care and consideration for other people.

"But speaking the truth in love, we must grow up in every way into Him who is the head, into Christ."
Ephesians 4:15

Godly speaking involves both parts: truth and love. When we neglect one part in our conversation we risk doing harm. Truth without love is too harsh. Love without truth rings hollow.

Jesus always spoke the truth with love. That's why amazed listeners declared, "No man ever spoke like this Man!" (John 7:46). That's why thousands gathered to hear Him, clinging to His words.

He is the living Word — love and truth with skin on them. As we "grow up in every way into Him," we too will speak the truth in love.

IN YOUR OWN WORDS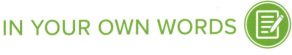

REPHRASE THE BIBLE'S ADVICE ON LANGUAGE MATTERS.

....

....

....

....

JESUS SUMS UP THE TWO MAIN POINTS TO LIFE

"One of the teachers of the law came and heard them debating. Noticing that Jesus had given them a good answer, he asked Him, 'Of all the commandments, which is the most important?' 'The most important one,' answered Jesus, 'is this: "Hear, O Israel, the Lord our God, the Lord is one. Love the Lord your God with all your heart and with all your soul and with all your mind and with all your strength." 'The second is this: "Love your neighbor as yourself." 'There is no commandment greater than these.'" Mark 12:28-31

Advice columnist Ann Landers put it this way: "If you have love in your life, it can make up for a great many things you lack. If you don't have it, no matter what else there is, it's not enough."

"Finally, all of you, have unity of spirit, sympathy, love for one another, a tender heart, and a humble mind." 1 Peter 3:8

To love God fully means we must genuinely love everyone. It is said, "We love God only as much as we love the person we love least."

This doesn't mean we have to *like* the person or what they do. It does mean we wish the best for them, desiring God's love and Spirit of integrity and peace to fill them as He has filled us. This love means we choose never to be dominated by fear or resentment; instead, in each of our relationships we seek truth and offer grace.

"Beloved, let us love one another, for love is of God; and everyone who loves is born of God and knows God. He who does not love does not know God, for God is love." 1 John 4:7, 8

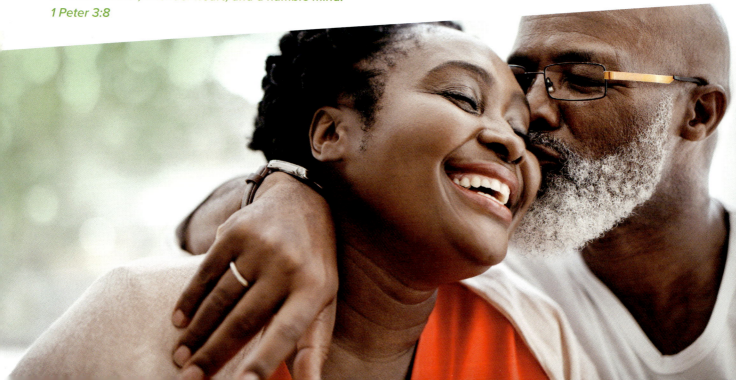

LIFE APPLICATION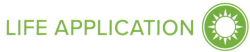

Take a moment to reflect on this study of interpersonal relationships.

WHAT PRINCIPLES HAVE YOU LEARNED THAT YOU WANT TO APPLY IN YOUR LIFE?

....

....

....

....

Examples of goals for interpersonal relationships:

My goal is to enjoy a date with my wife/husband once a week on this night: _____.

My goal each morning is to ask for God's help to control a hasty temper that damages my relationships.

My goal is to spend at least one hour a day with my children.

My goal is to be gracious to everybody each day — forgiving, accepting and sharing — as God has been gracious to me.

My goal is to respectfully consider the ideas my wife/husband shares with me, and not instantly squelch them.

NOW, CREATE A PERSONAL GOAL FOR STRENGTHENING YOUR INTERPERSONAL RELATIONSHIPS.

....

....

....

....

SMALL GROUP DISCUSSION QUESTIONS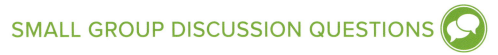

1. **FROM THE FIRST "HEAR THE HEARTBEAT" ACTIVITY, SHARE YOUR DESCRIPTION OF YOURSELF WHEN YOU ARE AUTHENTICALLY YOU.**

....

....

....

2. **WHICH STORY OR QUOTE DID YOU ESPECIALLY ENJOY?**

....

....

....

3. **DO YOU THINK "LOVE YOUR ENEMY" IS THE MOST RADICAL, COUNTERCULTURAL COMMAND OF ANY RELIGION? WHAT WOULD HAPPEN IF CHRISTIANS TOOK THIS COMMAND SERIOUSLY?**

....

....

....

The apples surest to go bad are those that never get out of the barrel. Susan Doenim

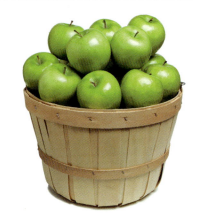

4. OF THE THREE PARTS OF GRACE — FORGIVING, ACCEPTING, AND SHARING —
    WHICH DO YOU APPRECIATE MOST? WHY?

....

....

....

5. WHAT LEVEL OF COMMUNICATION DO YOU THINK WE HAVE REACHED IN OUR GROUP?

....

....

....

6. SHARE A BIBLE TEXT THAT INSPIRED YOU.

....

....

....

7. COMMUNICATE ONE INTERPERSONAL GOAL WITH THE GROUP.
    HOW COULD OUR GROUP HELP YOU WITH THIS?

....

....

....

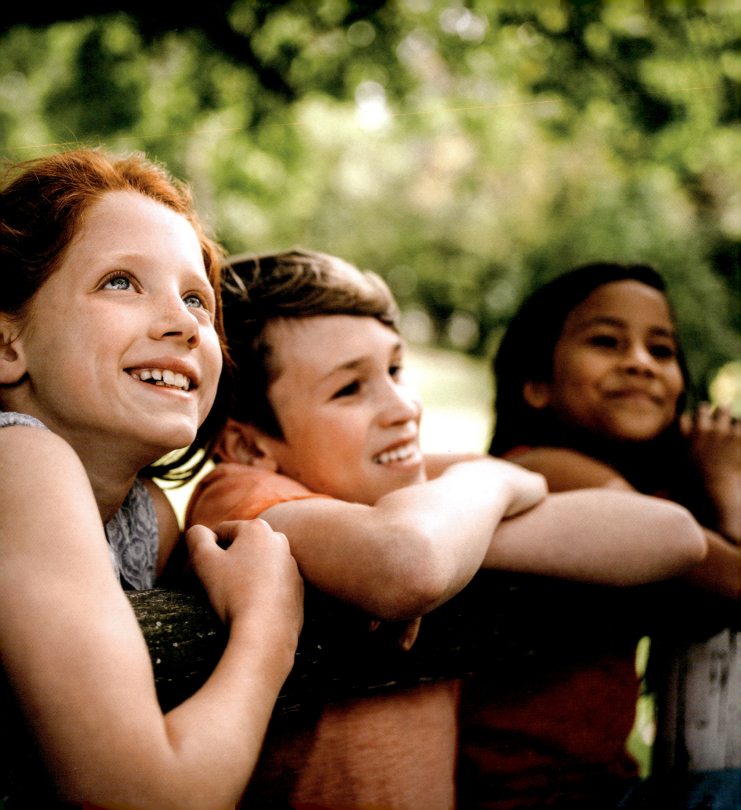

OUTLOOK

For I know the thoughts that I think toward you, says the Lord, thoughts of peace and not of evil, to give you a future and a hope. *Jeremiah 29:11*

Once there was a small mountain village nestled next to a high cliff. The happy villagers spent their days filled with laughter and activity much of the time, but an unsettling problem hung like a dark cloud over everyone. Again and again, one of the village children would wander off alone to the cliff only to slip and fall over the side. By the time the victim could be reached, it was too late.

The villagers held a meeting to find a solution. After hearing stories from grieving relatives and friends expressing their anguish and frustration, a plan was formed. Because the victims couldn't be reached in time to save their lives, a path would need to be built, winding to the base of the cliff. Then someone asked if the injured could be properly transported back to the village. Obviously, a vehicle would make the safest rescue.

It was decided the vehicle should be an ambulance, and the ambulance ought to have a trained, paid attendant, as well as a driver. They must be on call 24 hours a day because accidents can happen at any time. Figuring it out, they concluded at least six trained people should be housed in the ambulance service station — which, of course, they would have to build first.

Then came the question of funding. Who would pay for it all? They determined taxes would have to be raised and revenues collected to open a rescue training school within the village. Of course, the tuition would help to pay for the instructors, administrators, utilities and upkeep of the grounds.

After much discussion and planning, and realizing the enormous expenses and staggering sacrifices called for — in the midst of an argument over which make of ambulance got the best gas mileage on mountains — an ancient great-grandfather struggled to his feet and asked one poignant question.

"Why don't you put up a fence?"

In 1903, Thomas Edison wrote, "The doctor of the future will give no medicine, but will instruct his patient in the care of the human frame, in diet and in the cause and prevention of disease." In ancient China, the doctor got paid only if the patient stayed well.

How we see the world and what we choose to focus on is a crucial element of CREATION Life. We call this focus "outlook," and as the villagers in the story found out, it determines our course of action in any given situation.

Which health approach will you take — the fence or the ambulance?

Where I Am (Place a mark on the line to show what you're feeling right now.)

My outlook tends to be gloomy with scattered showers.

My outlook is sunny with radiant hope and joy.

I believe in Christianity as I believe in the sun — not only because I can see it, but because by it I can see everything else. C. S. Lewis

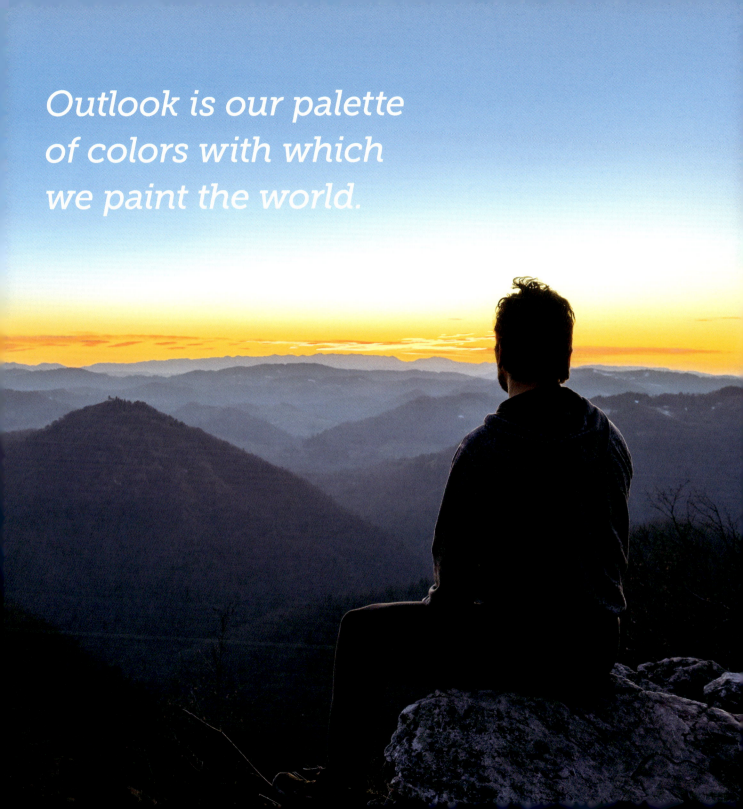

Outlook is our palette of colors with which we paint the world.

Everything good was offered by God as an enduring gift at Creation. But when we separated from God, the human prospect soured like a carton of curdled milk. Fortunately, we can reclaim what was lost. A realistic outlook begins with an honest appraisal of our true condition.

King Frederick II, an Eighteenth-Century king of Prussia, was visiting a prison in Berlin when he discovered honesty is hard to come by. One by one, the inmates tried to convince him that they had been framed, duped and unjustly imprisoned. Amid their protests of innocence, the king spotted one man sitting alone in a corner, oblivious to the commotion. When the king asked the man what he was there for, the prisoner replied, "Armed robbery, your Honor."

The king asked, "Were you guilty?"

"Yes, sir," he answered. "I entirely deserve my punishment."

The king quickly issued an order. "Release this guilty man! I don't want him corrupting all these innocent people."

"All we like sheep have gone astray; we have turned, every one, to his own way; and the Lord has laid on Him the iniquity of us all." Isaiah 53:6

Many people are unaware they are lost. Many more don't know they are found. When we discover we are truly forgiven and accepted by God, it brings the freedom we so desperately seek. And it also brings something else: eternal joy.

"These things I have spoken to you, that My joy may remain in you, and that your joy may be full." John 15:11

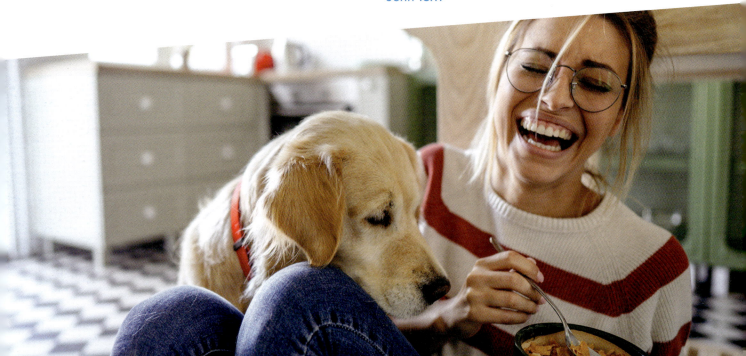

In South Africa, a pastor met a woman who radiated joy. She was confined to a wheelchair, and her hands were badly disfigured. Years earlier, she had contracted leprosy, and while she was in the leprosarium terrible tragedies hit. Her only son died of polio, her husband succumbed to cancer and a sister was killed in an automobile crash.

One day while placing drops in the woman's eyes, a nurse accidentally put in carbolic acid. This destroyed the woman's eyesight. Not long after, gangrene necessitated the amputation of one leg. During the first 55 years of her life she had 56 operations.

Yet how did she react to this avalanche of tragedy? Did she complain about her misfortunes or the unfairness of it all? Quite the opposite. She talked of her blessings, the goodness of God and all He had done for her. This was no pretense. Her glowing face confirmed every word.

How is it possible to carry a positive outlook in the face of such immense difficulties? Only by maintaining the assurance that God deeply cares about us and will bring His gracious goodness upon us.

"Jesus wept. Then the Jews said, 'see how He loved him!'" John 11:35, 36

Helen Keller, who endured more than her share of troubles, wrote, "Self-pity is our worst enemy, and if we yield to it we can never do anything wise in the world. Life is an exciting business, and most exciting when it is lived for others."

"Do all things without complaining or arguing." Philippians 2:14

REMEMBER THIS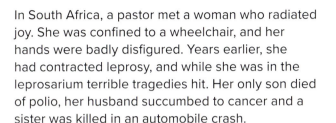

One way to focus on the good in life is to memorize Bible promises and meditate on them.

WRITE A NEW BIBLE PROMISE YOU WANT TO COMMIT TO MEMORY TO HELP YOU THROUGH THE CHALLENGES OF LIFE.

....

....

....

....

....

....

....

Joy is the most infallible sign of the presence of God.

Leon Bly

SELF-SERVING BIAS

"Every way of a man is right in his own eyes, but the Lord weighs the hearts."   *Proverbs 21:2*

We tend to judge ourselves more generously than we judge others. Social scientists label this tendency *self-serving bias*. When others mess up, their personal defects are to blame, but when we have problems, the explanations exist outside ourselves.[1]

"THEY"

- Didn't listen well
- Weren't trying hard enough
- Were angry, out of control
- Are moody and oversensitive
- Should have been more careful

"I"

- Received unclear directions
- Didn't have enough time
- Needed to "blow off steam"
- Have been under a lot of pressure
- Couldn't really avoid it

Biased perceptions lead to "outlook blindness." In one study, a random sample of men ranked themselves on their ability to get along with others.[2] Every person placed himself in the top half of the population. Further defying the laws of probability, 60 percent rated themselves in the top 10 percent, and 25 percent believed they were in the top 1 percent!

In his book *Everything but Money*, Sam Levenson recalls how a poor home with immigrant parents worked against self-serving bias.

> I didn't know I had to *feel like* doing my homework, practicing the violin, washing dishes or running errands. I just had to do it because everyone had to do things he really didn't feel like doing — even big people. I had a strong suspicion my father didn't feel like working 12 hours a day in a sweatshop.

> As an additional safeguard against self-pity in our home, Mama kept several charity boxes marked "For the Poor." We gave regularly. It made us feel rich.

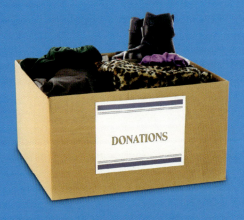

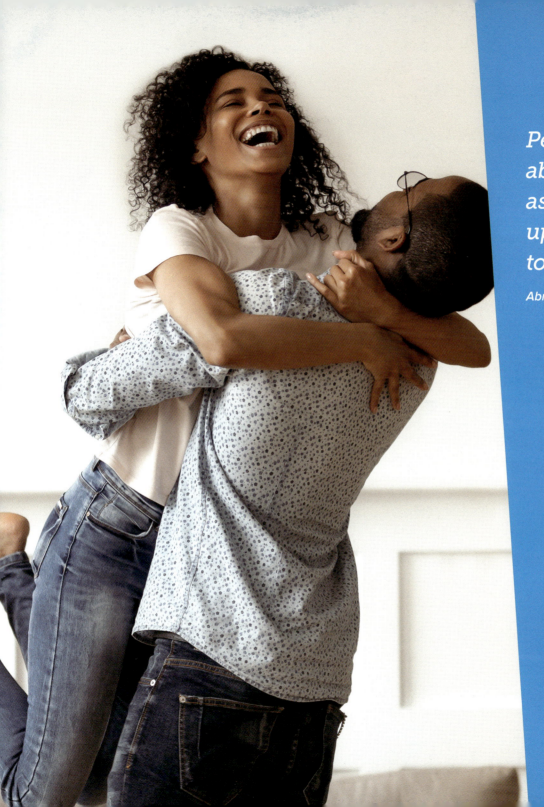

People are about as happy as they make up their minds to be.

Abraham Lincoln

WE BELIEVE WHAT WE DO

Psychologist Leon Festinger reached the conclusion that *we believe what we do more than we do what we believe*. That is, if you do something enough you come to believe it. This principle runs counter to schooling which focuses on enabling students to believe a truth first. But "cognitive dissonance" dictates we cannot continue to do something and persist in believing it's wrong. Instead, we tend to rationalize: *Oh, it's okay this once. Everybody does it anyway. I deserve this. Probably nobody will get hurt.*

That's why it's so important to make a habit of doing the right things. It's also why teenagers can sit unmoved through 60 sermons on the importance of Christian service, yet one mission trip changes their entire outlook. They come to believe it by doing it.

Naturally, Jesus understood this basic law of the human mind:

"For where your treasure is, there your heart will be also." Matthew 6:21

Our "treasure" is our time, our assets and our energies. Wherever we choose to invest ourselves, we trust the deposit. As Fred Smith notes,

> God is basically interested not in our money but in our maturity. Some people try to substitute service for giving, while others give to avoid serving. Neither one works; both are required for Christian maturity. That's why if you show me your calendar and your checkbook, I can write your biography. I will know how you spend your time and your money; that constitutes your treasure.

Our outlook is constructed one action and thought at a time, yet the accrued results can be beyond comprehension. In *Mere Christianity*, C. S. Lewis comments:

> Good and evil both increase at compound interest. That is why the little decisions you and I make every day are of such infinite importance. The smallest good act today is the capture of a strategic point from which, a few months later, you may be able to go on to victories you never dreamed of.

Those who in everything make God first and last and best are the happiest people in the world. Ellen White

"But we all, with unveiled face, beholding as in a mirror the glory of the Lord, are being transformed into the same image from glory to glory, just as by the Spirit of the Lord." 2 Corinthians 3:18

We become changed by beholding the glory of God, and that glory — the ultimate glory of self-sacrificing love — is seen most clearly in the person of Jesus. In the end, if we want a godly life free of self-serving bias, we must behold Jesus. Begin by reading the gospels — Matthew, Mark, Luke and John. Contemplate His courage, marvel at His unfailing compassion, witness His relentless friendship.

"Then Jesus came out, wearing the crown of thorns and the purple robe. And Pilate said to them, behold the Man!'" John 19:5

FOCAL POINT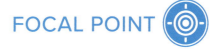

Have you invested enough time and energy in making a habit of looking closely at the life of Jesus?

I CAN INVEST _____ MINUTES LOOKING AT JESUS AT THIS TIME EVERY WEEK:

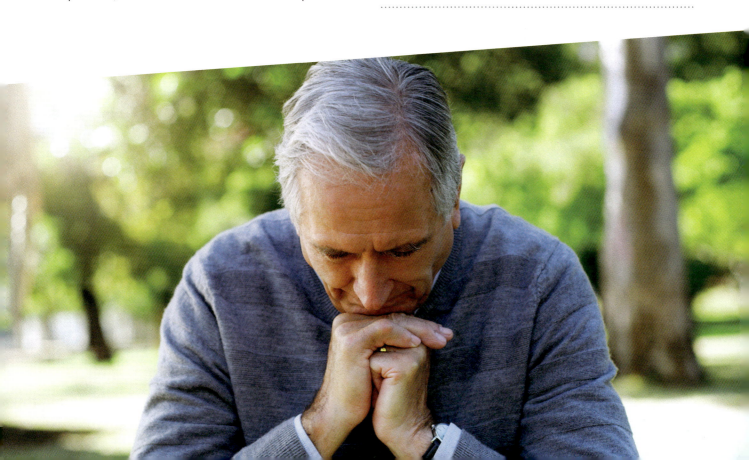

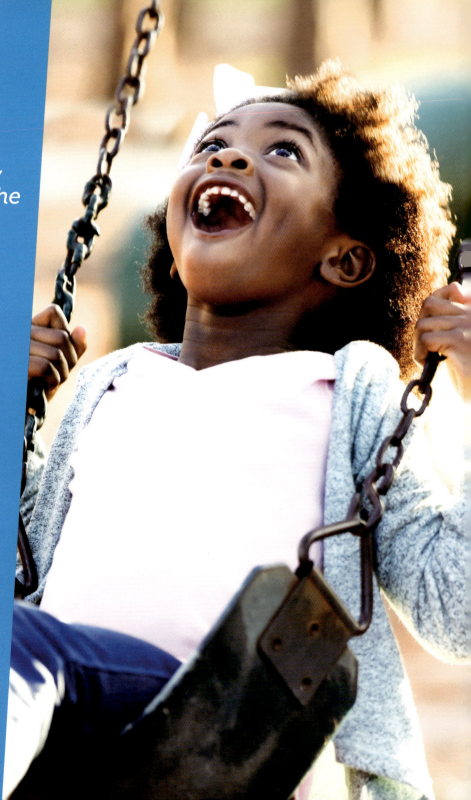

Whoever humbles himself like this child, he is the greatest in the kingdom of heaven.

Matthew 18:4

REQUIRER OR ASPIRER?

A vital outlook distinction emerges from asking ourselves one question: "Am I a requirer or an aspirer?"

Requirers demand that life be fair while insisting that their own wants are met. The requirer deals in commands and controls, making constant requirements of everyone and everything around them. Requirers insist that life be wonderfully fine, and when it's not, they respond with frustration, anger or blame.

Aspirers desire that life be fair, and they strive toward that end. The aspirers, however, recognize the fact that all of their wants cannot be met. They also realize that meeting all of their wants might not carry the ultimate good of all, and that's a key concern for them. They're satisfied with their balanced best even if the world isn't at its best. Aspirers aim at making the world better, and toward that end they accept, adapt, appreciate and act.

As an aspiring example, consider what space travelers went through flying largely at the mercy of their craft and innumerable factors outside of their control. Alan Shepard, one of the early astronauts, admitted, "It's a very sobering feeling to be up in space and realize that one's safety factor was determined by the lowest bidder on a government contract."

Yet those courageous explorers went *way* out of their comfort zone to push the boundaries of human knowledge and achievement. So can we.

LIFE APPLICATION

Becoming an aspirer means we have to let go of the demands of our ego. Dr. Wayne Dyer offers seven steps for overcoming ego's hold:

1. Stop being offended.

2. Let go of your need to win.

3. Let go of your need to be right.

4. Let go of your need to be superior.

5. Let go of your need to have more.

6. Let go of identifying yourself on the basis of your achievements.

7. Let go of your reputation.

CIRCLE AND THEN WRITE DOWN THE NUMBER/S YOU NEED TO RELINQUISH.

....

....

Have nothing to do with stupid, senseless controversies; you know that they breed quarrels.

2 Timothy 2:23

ATTITUDE OF GRATITUDE

"Oh, give thanks to the Lord, for He is good! For His mercy endures forever." Psalm 136:1

Carrying an attitude of gratitude always improves outlook. Gratitude releases ego's hold on us. You can express your thanks to God for the breath of life filling your lungs, for the blessings of life flooding your very existence.

An outlook marked by anxiety is an endless disaster. The story is told of a woman on a cruise ship who was an extremely nervous traveler; she was constantly running to the captain with her fears. When the ship finally came to its destination, the captain said to her, "You can stop worrying now, madam. We've dropped the anchor."

"I'm not surprised," the woman said. "It's been hanging over the side for days."

"I will praise the name of God with a song, and will magnify Him with thanksgiving." Psalm 69:30

The impact of gratefulness was a topic of researchers Emmons and McCullough. They asked three groups to keep a weekly journal recording various features. One group recorded items they were grateful for. Another reported neutral events. The last detailed their problems.

At the end of the study, the results were obvious. The group that kept track of items for which they were grateful exercised more regularly, reported fewer physical illness symptoms, were more optimistic and felt prepared for the upcoming days.[3] Having an attitude of gratitude truly does affect our health.

LIFE APPLICATION

WHO COULD YOU EXPRESS YOUR GRATITUDE TO TODAY, AND FOR WHAT REASON?

NAME:

....

....

REASON:

....

....

....

"The light of the eyes rejoices the heart, and a good report makes the bones healthy." Proverbs 15:30

GRATITUDE JOURNAL:
Each night, write down three things you were grateful for during the day. Express your thanksgiving to God and others for these blessings. This is a sure way to brighten your outlook.

POSITIVELY FOCUSED

Mountain bikers sometimes encounter large rocks in the middle of a single-track path. If they concentrate on the rock, they hit it and take a tumble. But experienced bikers learn to focus on a route *beside* the obstacle. This allows them to miss the rock and keep going.

Our focus should be on the good and true, noble and pure. This doesn't mean we never experience a sad thought or feel angry about injustice, but we don't get mired in these modes — we remain agile. Through a positive outlook we learn to adjust and move on with life, knowing that in the end God will make all things right.

If we focus on past hurts, we become bitter. If we focus on frustrations, we become irritable. If we focus on grievances, we become hateful. In his book *Love, Acceptance, and Forgiveness*, Jerry Cook comments on this perspective.

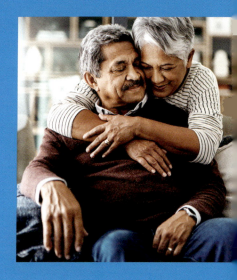

"And now, my friends, all that is true, all that is noble, all that is just and pure, all that is lovable and gracious, whatever is excellent and admirable — fill all your thoughts with these things." Philippians 4:8

> I've seen husbands and wives live together as though they were vultures. He's perched over here and she's perched over there and they meet in an arena between. Each is just waiting for the other to make a mistake so he or she can lash out. Have you learned yet that people tend to live up to your expectations of them? Just perch there watching for your husband or wife to blow it again and you probably won't have to wait too long.

> "My husband is never on time for anything," a woman said to me. "And he is always in a bad mood. He has never been able to handle money either." She went down a list of about 15 things that her husband "always" or "never" did.

> When she finished I said, "You undoubtedly have the most consistent husband I've ever heard of. You have been married for 24 years and this guy has made totally wrong decisions all that time — quite a record."

> You get the point and so did she. What are you looking for? You will find it.

The good news is that by focusing on the positive qualities in others, our lives begin demonstrating these qualities as well. When we focus on finding love, we become more loving. When we focus on finding mercy, we become compassionate. When we focus on finding blessings, we become grateful.

RE-EVALUATING YOUR CAN'TS

"And my God shall supply all your needs according to His riches in glory by Christ Jesus." Philippians 4:19

A self-fulfilling prophecy means our low expectations of an event make the outcome more likely to occur. Fearful people often assume what social scientists term the fallacy of catastrophic expectations: the belief that if something bad can possibly happen, it will. (Note that this is an official fallacy). This self-talk influences our outlook, actions and the quality of our life. We literally "psych" ourselves out.

SAMPLE STATEMENTS:

"I can't talk about important things with my family."

"I can't ask my boss questions."

"I can't be myself with people I'd like to get to know."

"I can't stop criticizing my friend."

The future is not what it used to be.

Paul Valery

Take two minutes right now to address your self-talk. Simply list the statements you typically say that begin with "I can't… " Focus on your relationships with family, friends, co-workers and strangers.

1. **I CAN'T**
....
2. **I CAN'T**
....
3. **I CAN'T**
....

Now, cross out each *can't* and change it to *won't*. How does this make you feel? Analyze why you won't take these actions. What are you afraid of? Could internal voices be holding you back?

Take those statements and refocus what you can do in these areas.

1. **I CAN**
....
2. **I CAN**
....
3. **I CAN**
....

Feel free to write out an expanded list of *I cans* and refer to it often. Soon your outlook will be more focused on what you *can* do.

"Fear not, for I am with you; be not dismayed, for I am your God. I will strengthen you, yes, I will help you." Isaiah 41:10

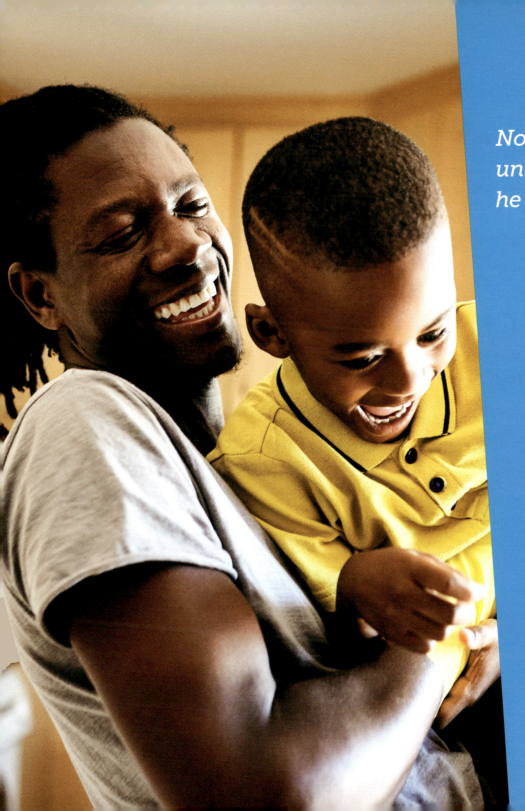

No man is happy unless he believes he is. **Publilius Syrus**

CREATE OPPORTUNITY

Sometimes people become too rigid in their righteousness. We can stick to our principles and also stay flexible with a creative approach. Pastor Earl Palmer tells a story that illustrates all three of these traits.

A Christian friend of mine was a high school principal in Los Angeles. One day a father came charging into his office, irate over the F his son had received in a certain course. The man had dreams of his son going to an Ivy League school, and now this teacher was destroying the plan. The father wanted the grade changed.

My friend listened to the threats and demands for a while, and finally when there was a pause, he said quietly, "I can see that you care a great deal about your son."

The man suddenly began to cry. The mask came off. He was strong but aloof, and the only way he knew how to do anything for his son was by bullying. When the principal spoke about their relationship, the point of deepest hurt was exposed. Now the father was ready to be helped.

My friend knew he wasn't going to ask the teacher to change the grade. So why be defensive? Instead, he listened with his heart until he got in touch with the man's underlying journey.

"In the beginning God created." Genesis 1:1

Fortunately, after Creation, God kept on creating right along with His creations. Think of the many ways our adaptable God turns problems into opportunities:

Problem: Human children rebel and start acting out of fear

Opportunity: Send a loving Savior to rescue them

Problem: The temple sanctuary — God's house — is destroyed

Opportunity: Establish a sacred sanctuary within each person

Problem: So many differences between different people

Opportunity: Change differences into strengths — unity in diversity

"Behold, I will do a new thing. Now it shall spring forth; shall you not know it?" Isaiah 43:19

IN YOUR OWN WORDS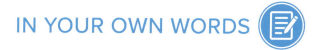

Follow God's creative lead and adapt a few issues in your life. How can these become opportunities?

PROBLEM

A.
....

....

B.
....

....

C.
....

....

OPPORTUNITY

A.
....

....

B.
....

....

C.
....

....

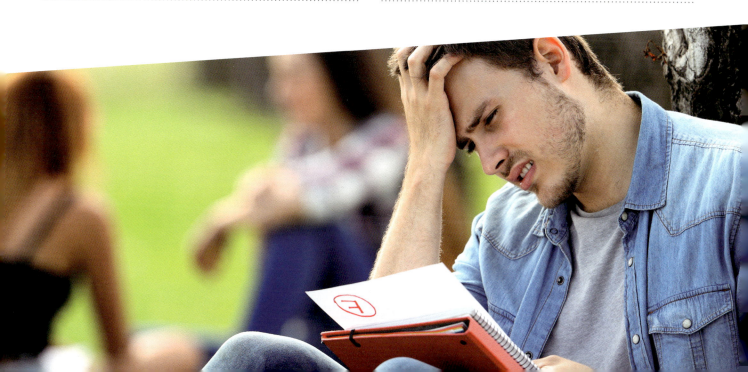

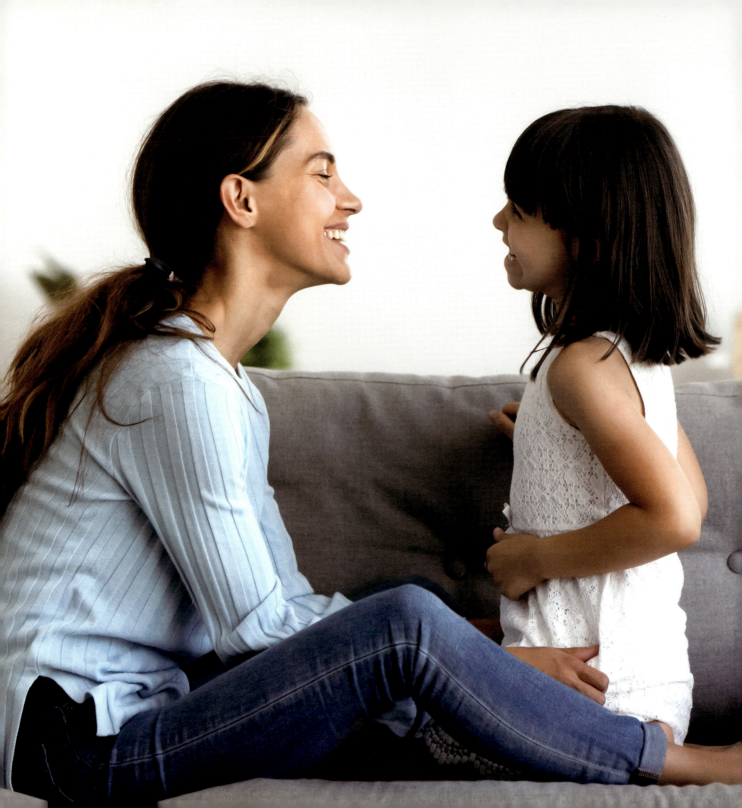

LIVING ON PURPOSE

"One thing I do, forgetting those things which are behind and reaching forward to those things which are ahead, I press toward the goal for the prize of the upward call of God in Christ Jesus."
Philippians 3:13, 14

Clear vision gives us a goal to work toward while fresh purpose furnishes us with a reason to live. When we are struggling to take one more step, we can envision a brighter future and gather courage to persevere.

In his essay, "The Future-Focused Role Image," Benjamin Singer indicates that "low-performance students had almost no sense of their future. Their focus was strictly short term." These children believed their future was entirely in the hands of fate and out of their control.

However, successful students carried a much greater sense of control over their future; they thought in horizons of five to ten years out. When identifying successful students, IQ and family background were not key indicators of success. Instead, successful students shared a purposeful and positive vision of their future.[4]

When your children talk of what they will be, take their thoughts seriously. Help them make their vision a reality.

"There is hope in your future, says the Lord, that your children shall come back to their own border."
Jeremiah 31:17

LIFE APPLICATION

Take time this week to write your personal mission statement. What is your reason for existence? Start with a few chosen thoughts right now. Keep a copy of your statement in your wallet to remind you at all times. Consider asking your children to create a personal statement for themselves.

PERSONAL MISSION STATEMENT

....

....

....

What is a purposeful vision for your family? Gather your family together to draft a statement of your family's values. Could our children benefit from more specifics than "Love God and keep your room clean?"

Ask each family member for input — perhaps five essential traits — and combine them into one statement. When everyone is agreed on the final product, frame and post it in a visible spot in your home.[5]

OUR FAMILY VALUES

1.
....
2.
....
3.
....
4.
....
5.
....

JESUS' MISSION AND VISION

"The Spirit of the Lord God is upon Me, because the Lord has anointed Me to preach good tidings to the poor; He has sent Me to heal the brokenhearted, to proclaim liberty to the captives, and the opening of the prison to those who are bound." Luke 4:18, 19

Though constantly hounded by the religious leaders of His day, Jesus kept right on fighting because of His purpose (which included all of us today). His mission was always front and center in His thinking and continually propelled Him forward. Even to difficult and dark places.

"For the joy that was set before Him [Jesus] endured the cross, despising the shame, and has sat down at the right hand of the throne of God." Hebrews 12:2

Jesus' joyful vision and commitment carried Him through it all. He maintained a broader, deeper, longer outlook because He knew, and knows, what we can only imagine. The prophet Elisha also knew.

"And when the servant of the man of God arose early and went out, there was an army, surrounding the city with horses and chariots. And his servant said to him, 'Alas, my master! What shall we do?' So [Elisha] answered, 'Do not be afraid, for those who are with us are greater than those who are with them.' And Elisha prayed, and said, 'Lord, I pray, open his eyes that he may see.' Then the Lord opened the eyes of the young man, and he saw. And behold, the mountain was full of horses and chariots of fire all around Elisha." 2 Kings 6:15-17

Life is more than what we can see with our eyes — there are unseen realities. If this is difficult to imagine, think about the unseen qualities of x-rays and gamma rays, gravity and wind, protons and electrons — yet we can "see" their impact.

But there are other dimensions just as real. We are surrounded by a bristling universe, an unseen battlefield of spiritual warfare fighting for the trusting allegiance of all of the earth's inhabitants.

On one side, the enemy of souls employs deception and coercion: the marks of the beast. On the opposing side, the Creator wields truth and love. The greatest casualty in this war was the Son of God, who endured the cross. Paradoxically, the greatest victor in the war is the Son of God, who for the joy set before Him arose from the dead and reigns forevermore. May we look at life as He sees it.

Lord, open our eyes to see You at work in the unseen.

HUMBLE ASSURANCE

Too often, Christians lack humble assurance. They strain to believe that they are, in fact, children of the Most High God, the King of Kings. One of the saddest things in the world is a Christian who is "just not sure if God loves them." With this in mind, let's examine several texts that make plain God's outlook on salvation.

"For the righteous fall seven times and rise again; but the wicked are overthrown by calamity." Proverbs 24:16

Do you see the main difference between the righteous and the wicked? The righteous keep getting up! Look at it this way: Let's say you walk into an elevator and punch the button for the top floor. On the ride up, you lose your balance and take a fall in the elevator. You may be embarrassed or upset, but here's the good news: *You're still headed up.*

Fallen and resilient, our outlook is found in the rising, eternal light of the Cross and Resurrection of Jesus. As Jesus, Peter, Paul and John put it:

"I am the resurrection and the life. Those who believe in me, even though they die, will live." John 11:25

"It shall be that whoever calls on the name of the Lord shall be saved." Acts 2:21

"I am sure that he who began a good work in you will bring it to completion at the day of Jesus Christ." Philippians 1:6

"These things I have written to you who believe in the name of the Son of God, that you may know that you have eternal life." 1 John 5:13

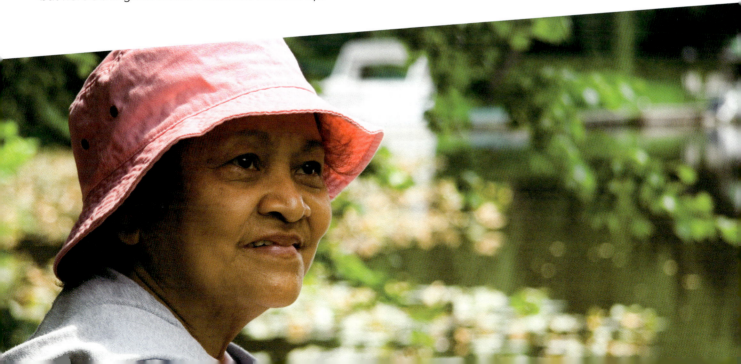

Will *live*. *Shall* be saved. I am *sure*. That you may *know*. These are not wavering and cringing expressions of weak and crumbly trust. Look at these texts. All of them boldly declare *rock-solid* promise, security and support in the strongest possible language.

What sort of parent keeps a child insecure about whether the child is in the family? Imagine: "Are you really my mommy and daddy? I know you told me so a thousand times, but I disobeyed you just now, so I'm not really sure."

Only a sadistic parent would keep a child that fearful. Do we understand how we hurt God when we say this?

"Because of the increase of lawlessness, the love of many will grow cold. But the one who endures to the end will be saved." Matthew 24:12, 13

We cannot let our love grow cold. The enduring struggle we must face is to keep our eyes on Jesus, to see God as He truly is.

"Dear friends, now we are children of God, and what we will be has not yet been made known. But we know that when Christ appears, we shall be like Him, for we shall see Him as He is." 1 John 3:2

"I know that you are a gracious and merciful God, slow to anger and abundant in loving kindness, One who relents from doing harm." Jonah 4:2

"Personal salvation" doesn't begin in heaven or the new earth. The root of "salvation" is "salve" — a healing application. Salvation begins now. Think about the words used to describe life with God. *Everlasting* describes the duration — how long it lasts. *Eternal* is about quality of life — a deep, fearless, joyful friendship with God. Salvation is not the end of our life with Christ. It's the beginning.

That's why eternal life begins now. We are saved now. We are liberated from sin, from unresolved guilt and worry *now*.

Do you recall the story of Zacchaeus? Do you remember what Jesus said to His tree-climbing friend?

"Today, salvation has come to this house." Luke 19:9

For a healthy outlook today, repeat these eight words: *"Jesus has saved me. Jesus saves me now."*

Believe them every moment of every day. You are saved by His grace. So live with humble assurance every day of your life.

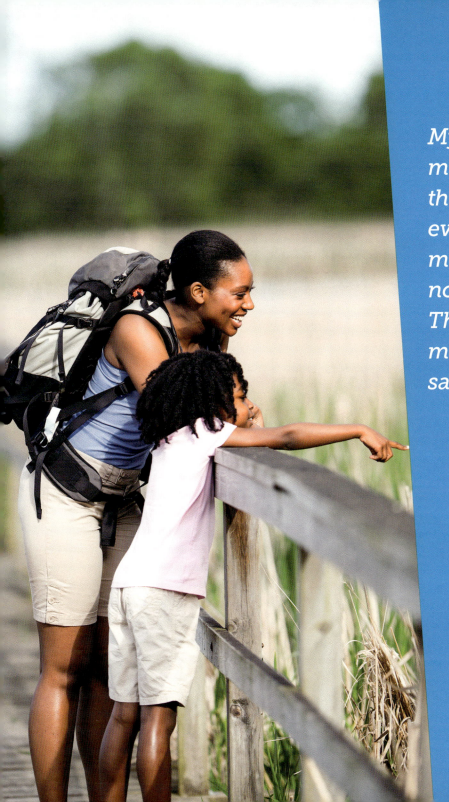

My Prayer: God, help me maintain an outlook that positively influences everyone I touch. Enable me to rely on the fence, not the ambulance. Thank You for granting me the assurance of Your salvation in my life.

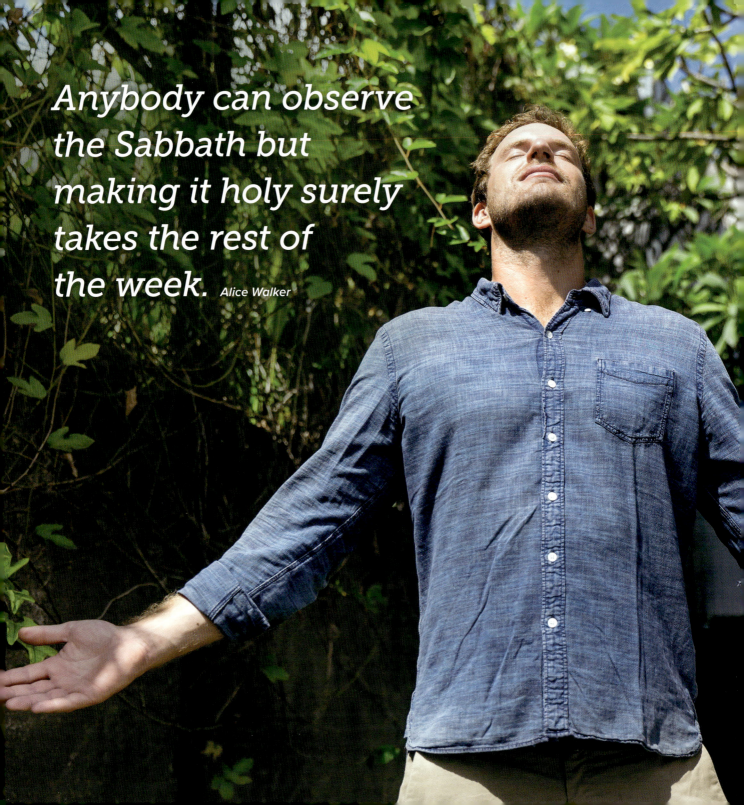

Anybody can observe the Sabbath but making it holy surely takes the rest of the week. Alice Walker

LIFE APPLICATION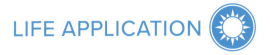

Take a moment to reflect on this CREATION Life study on outlook.

WHAT PRINCIPLES HAVE YOU LEARNED THAT YOU WANT TO APPLY IN YOUR LIFE?

....

....

....

....

....

....

NOW, CREATE A PERSONAL GOAL FOR YOUR OUTLOOK ON LIFE.

....

....

....

....

....

Examples of goals for outlook:

My goal is to thank someone at least once every day, and at night write three things I am thankful for from that day.

My goal is to identify a self-serving bias of mine and recognize it each time it rears its head for the next three weeks.

My goal is to stop saying "I can't" and start saying "I can."

My goal is to write a personal vision statement within the next week.

My goal is in two weeks to have my family agree on a statement of "Our Family Values."

My goal is to repeat eight words ("Jesus has saved me. Jesus saves me now") every time I feel afraid, enraged or tempted.

SMALL GROUP DISCUSSION QUESTIONS

1. HOW CAN THE PARABLE OF THE FENCE OR THE AMBULANCE BE APPLIED TO OUR PRACTICAL LIVES?

....
....
....

2. WHAT STORY OR ACTIVITY DID YOU ESPECIALLY APPRECIATE?

....
....
....

3. WHAT SELF-SERVING BIAS BOTHERS YOU MOST? WHICH ONE DO YOU MOST TEND TOWARD?

....
....
....

4. WHY DON'T WE SPEND MORE TIME LOOKING AT THE LIFE OF JESUS? IS IT REALLY THAT BIG A DEAL?

....
....
....

5. WHICH BIBLE TEXT HERE MEANS THE MOST TO YOU?

....

....

....

6. SHARE AN OUTLOOK GOAL. HOW AS A GROUP CAN WE HELP YOU WITH THIS GOAL?

....

....

....

7. IN WHAT WAY DID YOUR OUTLOOK CHANGE AS A RESULT OF THIS LESSON?

....

....

....

A saint is one who makes goodness attractive.

Laurence Housman

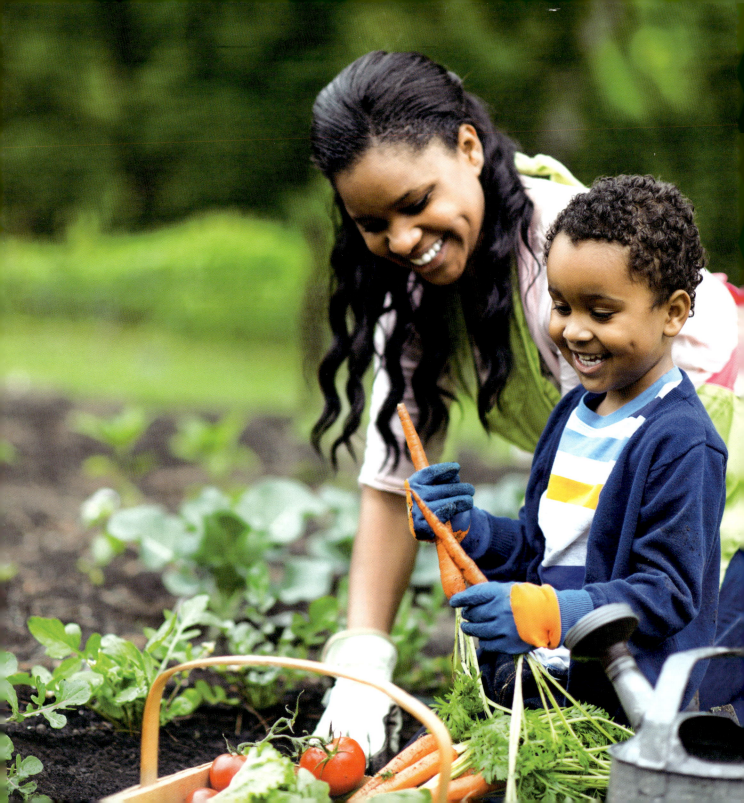

NUTRITION

Jesus said to them, "They do not need to go away. You give them something to eat." Matthew 14:16

Nutrition is simply the foods and nutrients we choose to put into our bodies. In the beginning, the Creator gave humanity a perfect diet for us to enjoy balanced, liberated lives. Somehow, though, we became captives to our lack of willpower. Dave Wilkinson uses a vivid account to illustrate this uncomfortable truth.

Thomas Costain's history, *The Three Edwards,* describes the life of Raynald III, a fourteenth-century duke in what is now Belgium. Grossly overweight, Raynald was commonly called by his Latin nickname, Crassus, which means "fat."

After a violent quarrel, Raynald's younger brother Edward led a successful revolt against him. Edward captured Raynald, but did not kill him. Instead, he built a room around Raynald in the Nieuwkerk castle and promised him he could regain his title and property as soon as he was able to leave the room.

This would not have been difficult for most people as the room had several windows and a door of near-normal size, and none was locked and barred. The problem was Raynald's size. To regain his freedom, he needed to lose weight. But Edward knew his older brother, and each day he sent a variety of delicious foods. Instead of dieting his way out of prison, Raynald grew fatter.

When Duke Edward was accused of cruelty, he had a ready answer: "My brother is not a prisoner. He may leave when he so wills."

Raynald stayed in that room for ten years and wasn't released until after Edward died in battle. By then, his health was so ruined that he died within a year — a prisoner of his own appetite.

How many of us today are prisoners of appetite? Amazingly, we construct our own prisons ourselves. But there's realistic hope. Though we may have built destructive barriers over many decades, the way out is clear.

Where I Am *(Place a mark on the line to show what you're feeling right now.)*

My eating habits are really awful.

I am nutritionally balanced and healthy.

Fear less, hope more; eat less, chew more; whine less, breathe more; talk less, say more; hate less, love more; and all good things will be yours.

Swedish Proverb

THE EDEN DIET

"The Lord God planted a garden eastward in Eden, and there He put the man whom He had formed. And out of the ground the Lord God made every tree grow that is pleasant to the sight and good for food." Genesis 2:9

Look at the beautiful story of how good food started. God, the first gardener, lovingly planted it for us. As our Creator, God planned for us to eat from the vegetation, including the tree of life. The planet was our banquet table.

The original menu brimmed with hearty grains, such as barley and oats; seeds, such as sesame and sunflower; and luscious fruits, such as apples, oranges, mangoes and nuts like almonds and pistachios.

This diet provided all the protein, complex carbohydrates, vitamins and minerals humans needed to function optimally. Modern science now strongly supports the benefits of a plant-based diet. God knew from the beginning what was best for our bodies.

"And God said, "See, I have given you every herb that yields seed which is on the face of all the earth, and every tree whose fruit yields seed; to you it shall be for food." Genesis 1:29

A key factor of the Eden diet is fiber. Fiber helps form walls within plant foods. These walls surround the substances we term "nutrients." Fiber is largely the indigestible portion of the plant, and helps to move the contents of the body's colon as well as slow the absorption of sugar (which keeps blood sugars from rising too quickly). As an extra benefit, fiber provides us with that satisfied "full" feeling without adding excess calories. A diet high in fiber has proven to help prevent heart disease, cancer and diabetes. It can also lower cholesterol, reduce blood pressure and fuel the brain.[1]

Another important feature of the Eden diet is color. Rich and vibrant colors of fruit and vegetables are present because of flavonoids, carotenoids, phyto-nutrients and other antioxidants. Antioxidants help prevent cellular damage — the pathway for cancer, aging and a variety of diseases. The general rule is the richer the color, the more nutrients contained.

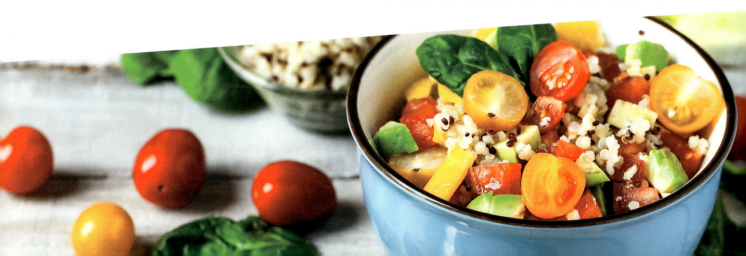

AS MUCH AS YOU NEED

"The drunkard and the glutton will come to poverty, and drowsiness will clothe a man with rags."
Proverbs 23:21

The word "glutton" refers to a person who overeats and seems to possess an insatiable appetite. Not only is overeating bad for us in terms of cholesterol, fat and uric acid, it also clouds our mind and makes us unproductive. Spacing our meals to provide time to properly digest each one helps us stay sharp. Between-meal snacks and beverages (except for water) keep the digestive cycle in constant motion, which drains our energy.

"Have you found honey? Eat only as much as you need." *Proverbs 25:16*

Researchers in the field of longevity have discovered one major common element in the lives of those who live a long time: They are often *light* eaters. Instead of ingesting large amounts of fat and calories throughout the day these individuals eat smaller, more focused meals to provide the energy they need. Healthy reduction could result in a huge impact on our lives.

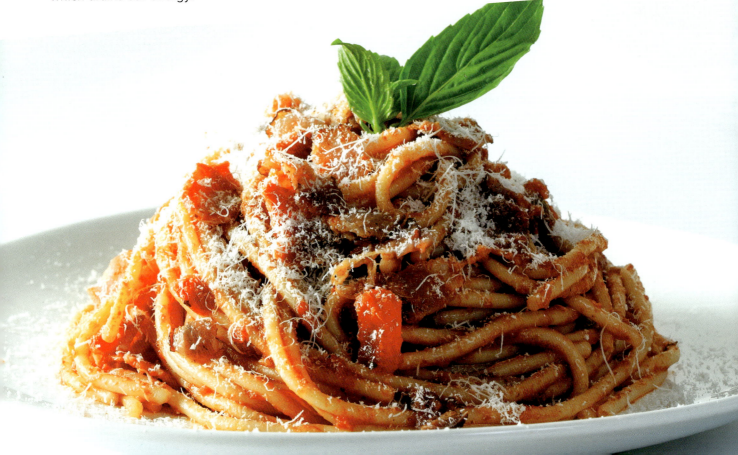

LIFE APPLICATION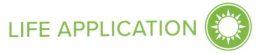

THINK OF THE REASONS OFFERED FOR OVEREATING.

(Check any you have used.)

- ☐ "WHEN I WAS A CHILD, I NEVER GOT ENOUGH TO EAT."
- ☐ "EATING IS HOW I HANDLE STRESS."
- ☐ "I LIKE FEELING FULL."
- ☐ "THE FOOD TASTED SO GOOD I COULDN'T STOP."
- ☐ "I DIDN'T THINK IT WAS POLITE TO TURN DOWN DESSERT — OR ANYTHING ELSE."
- ☐ "IT WAS SOMEBODY'S BIRTHDAY."
- ☐ "I WAS TAUGHT TO ALWAYS CLEAN MY PLATE."
- ☐ "IF I'M GOING TO PAY FOR IT, I'M GOING TO EAT IT."
- ☐ OTHER REASONS? *(WRITE BELOW)*

1. **WHAT MOTIVATES YOU TO EAT TOO MUCH?**

2. **DO YOU THINK THESE ARE RATIONAL, HELPFUL REASONS?**
   ☐ YES ☐ NO

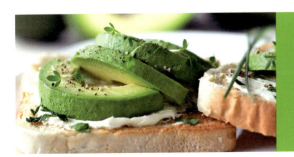

To lengthen thy life, lessen thy meals.

Benjamin Franklin

As a rule, the closer food remains to its original state the more nutritious it is. A baked or steamed whole potato retains more of its nutrients than processed tater tots, conveniently packaged for you in the freezer section and doused with preservatives, which barely resembles the original potato.

Whole grain foods are much healthier than foods that are mistakenly called "enriched." For example, a whole grain kernel of wheat contains 21 vitamins and minerals. A processed wheat kernel takes out the germ and bran. This strips the kernel of those 21 vitamins and minerals as well as most of the fiber. Then manufacturers put back only five of those vitamins, and call it "enriched." You are better off to eat the grain in its original package. Along with the label "organic" (which assures limited chemicals and toxins), look for the label "whole grain."

A wise consumer reads labels. By federal law, the closer an ingredient appears to the top of the ingredient list, the more of it is in the food. The fewer the ingredients on a label means the more natural the food is inside the package. And speaking of packaging, less is best — both for the environment and for our bodies. Food in less packaging has not been through many processes. Of course "natural" in the supermarket doesn't mean "direct from nature," as Bryan Francis points out.

Natural is not a legally standardized term, which basically means there is no government regulation for those foods. Everything can be classified as *natural*. Chemical waste, sewage sludge and conventional pesticides can all be considered *natural*. So please don't be fooled when you see the term *"natural"* being used to make a food look healthy. Food manufacturers and advertisers are geniuses in cashing in on the general public's ignorance, but I'm here to tell you that *"natural" Cheetos* are still *Cheetos*. When most people hear the term *natural*, they think of something occurring naturally on earth. Last time I checked, *Cheetos* don't grow from the ground or a tree.

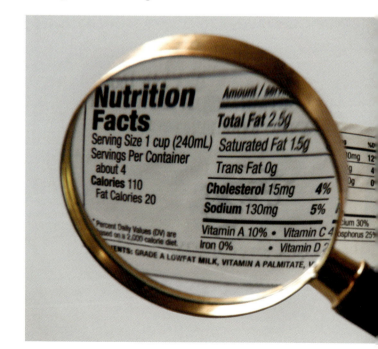

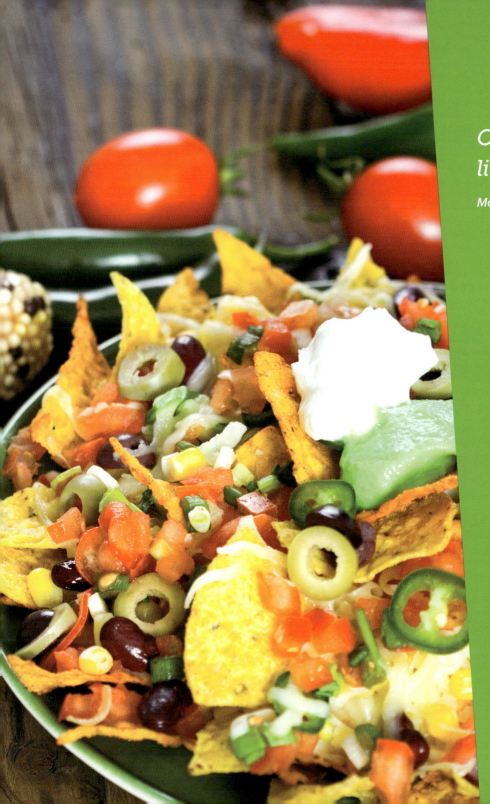

One must eat to live, not live to eat.

Moliere

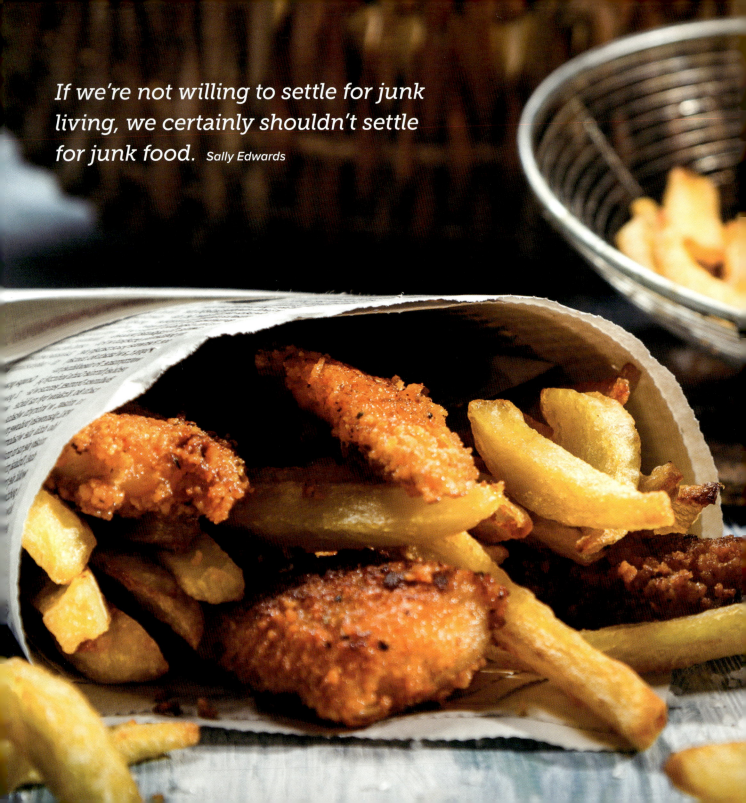

If we're not willing to settle for junk living, we certainly shouldn't settle for junk food. Sally Edwards

GOOD AND BAD FATS

"'If you diligently heed the voice of the Lord your God and do what is right in His sight, give ear to His commandments and keep all His statutes, I will put none of the diseases on you which I have brought on the Egyptians. For I am the Lord who heals you.'"
Exodus 15:26

A recent study on mummies determined that atherosclerosis, the disease caused by hardening of the arteries, was present thousands of years ago in ancient Egyptians. Those people didn't devour fast food or sit for hours watching high-definition TV. They had plenty of fresh air and exercise. However, they did eat meat, which is high in fat and cholesterol.[2]

"Then the whole congregation of the children of Israel complained against Moses and Aaron in the wilderness. And the children of Israel said to them, 'Oh, that we had died by the hand of the Lord in the land of Egypt, when we sat by the pots of meat and when we ate bread to the full!'"   Exodus 16:2, 3

God had led the Israelites out of slavery in Egypt, and had just miraculously provided sweet water in the desert for them, but the people were still angry. They missed their pot roast.

Not all fats are created equal. The fat found in meat is *saturated*, whereas the fats found in nuts, seeds and some fruits and vegetables, such as avocado, are *unsaturated*. While the body does need some fat, the fat it really needs is unsaturated, which lowers LDL (the bad) cholesterol levels. Saturated fats, found in meat and other animal products such as milk and cheese, raise LDL cholesterol levels.

EATING TOO LATE

Proper nutrition isn't just about what we eat — it's also important *when* we eat. Eating late can disturb our sleep (and dreams) because the body is still working to digest food. To enjoy restful, restorative sleep, go to sleep on an empty stomach, which means no eating during the three hours before bedtime.

At night as we sleep, our bodies are fasting, recovering from the previous day. By the morning, the body needs to be replenished to begin the new day. Breakfast literally means, "break the fast." Unfortunately in our society breakfast is frequently neglected, and when we do eat it, breakfast is often loaded with sugar, sodium and saturated fat. Studies find those who eat a healthy breakfast experience longer attention spans, more efficient problem solving, increased verbal fluency, more positive attitudes and better scholastic scores.[3]

When we are running around, working, keeping busy and not eating regularly, what happens? Our blood sugar drops. This can be a problem because when we get too hungry we are more prone to bingeing. We are also less likely to eat healthy foods. Pulling into a drive-thru or picking up a snack hanging inside the vending machine doesn't offer us the best choices.

Plan ahead if you have to be away from the table at mealtime. Keep some almonds, dried fruit or granola in a purse, desk or vehicle. These snacks can help you make healthier decisions about what you eat.

BENEFITS OF WATER

We now know the essential value of drinking water:

Assists in regulating body temperature

Carries nutrients and oxygen to cells

Allows joints to move smoothly

Helps the mind to think clearly

Cleans wastes from the body

Works as a natural diuretic

Aids in food digestion

Keeps skin flexible

Prevents fatigue

CHECK IT OUT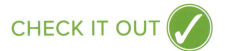

How many eight-ounce glasses of purified water do you drink each day?

☐ **9 OR MORE GLASSES**

☐ **7-8 GLASSES**

☐ **5-6 GLASSES**

☐ **3-4 GLASSES**

☐ **1-2 GLASSES**

The body is about 60 percent water and can survive only three days without receiving it. Dehydration is a serious condition that eventually causes the body's organs to shut down. The first signs of mild dehydration are headache, dizziness, reduced alertness and ability to concentrate, irritability and tiredness.

Did you notice something in the above list? *These are all common complaints.* Think about how many times you've heard individuals, or even yourself, complain about these ailments. Those symptoms can actually be a result of not drinking enough water. To maintain optimum health, drink at least eight eight-ounce glasses of purified water each day. To be quite candid, if your urine is not clear, you need more water. (That's "your analysis").

If you aren't intentional about drinking water, you likely aren't getting enough. Try carrying a refillable water bottle. Take advantage of the benefits of nature's best liquid.

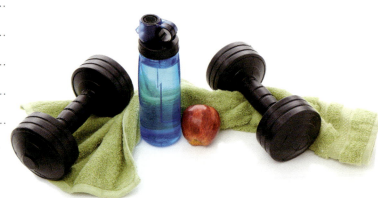

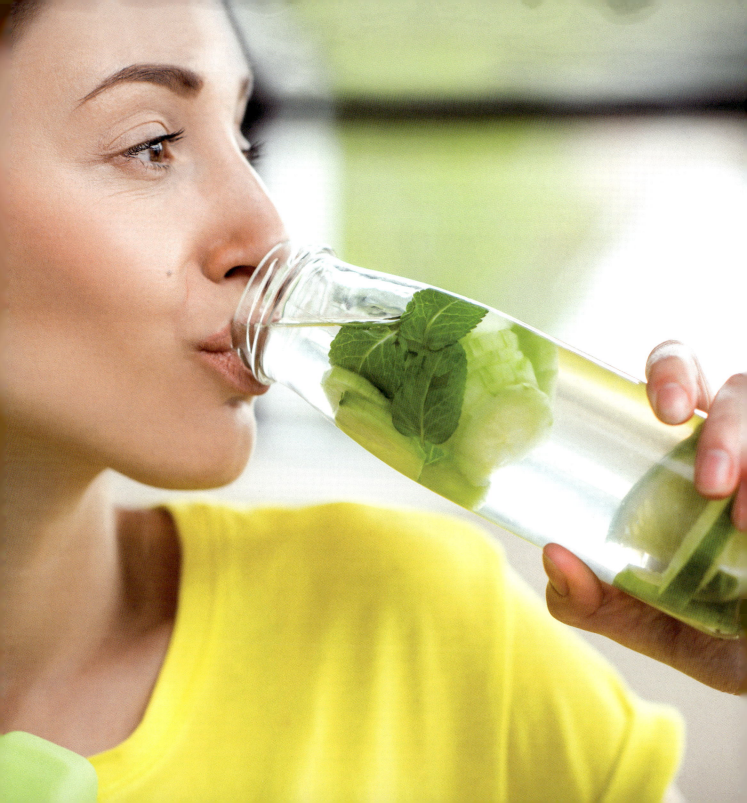

Though the Bible warns against drinking alcohol, advertisers and vendors want us to believe something else. "Alcohol isn't the problem," they say. "It is the abuse of alcohol by irresponsible or sick people that's the problem." Promoters even go so far as to portray alcohol as the key to enjoying a great party, dozens of hilarious friends and a blissful romantic life.

In reality, when confronted with decisions that must be made immediately such as driving, business, relationships and health, a mind clouded with alcohol might run a red light, engage in risky sexual behavior or create any number of regrettable life-altering mistakes.

In the United States, alcohol is a factor in about half of all human tragedies. One-half of all homicides, one-third of all suicides, one-half of all fatal car accidents, one-half of all rapes, 72 percent of all assaults (including spousal abuse), 70 percent of all robberies and one-half of all child-abuse cases are alcohol-related. Fetal alcohol exposure is the leading known cause of mental retardation.

Really, can we in good conscience support something that creates this much misery?

"Do not look on the wine when it is red, when it sparkles in the cup, when it swirls around smoothly; at the last it bites like a serpent, and stings like a viper. Your eyes will see strange things, and your heart will utter perverse things." Proverbs 23:31-33

FIVE WAYS TO SAY NO TO ALCOHOL

1. "I'm driving."

2. "I think I might be allergic to alcohol. It makes me really sick."

3. "No, thanks. I want to keep my head clear."

4. "I have an alcoholic in my family."

5. "I'd rather give you my full attention. Is that okay?"

I'd rather give you my full attention. Is that okay?

EFFECTS OF SMOKING

The Bible doesn't talk specifically about cigarettes, cigars or chewing tobacco, as tobacco was not commonly used in Bible times. However, we can deduce from the healthy nature of God that we ought to stay away from tobacco. Smoking is slow suicide.

Research is overwhelming on the devastating effects of tobacco on the human body. *Tobacco currently kills more people worldwide than HIV/AIDS, alcohol, drug abuse, fires, murders, suicides, drowning accidents and car crashes combined.* No business is more deadly than the tobacco industry. Consider these health facts:

- There is enough nicotine in five cigarettes to kill an average adult if ingested whole.

- Secondhand smoke contains more than 50 cancer-causing chemical compounds, including 11 Group 1 carcinogens.

- A typical cigarette contains 8 milligrams of nicotine, while the nicotine content of a typical cigar is 100 to 200 milligrams.

- Ambergris, otherwise known as whale vomit, is one of the hundreds of additives used in manufactured cigarettes.

- Half of all long-term smokers will die a tobacco-related death.

- Hydrogen cyanide, a toxic byproduct in cigarette smoke, was the lethal chemical used in Nazi gas chambers.

- Smoking can cause reproductive problems and sudden infant death syndrome.

- Worldwide, one in every five people age 13 to 15 smoke cigarettes.

- Approximately 25 percent of the youth alive today in the Western Pacific Region (East Asia and the Pacific) will die from tobacco use.[4]

In Australia, cigarette packs carry these warnings:

- Smoking causes blindness
- Smoking causes mouth and throat cancer
- Smoking harms unborn babies
- Smoking causes heart disease
- Smoking causes lung cancer
- Smoking doubles your risk of stroke

☐ **I WANT TO ELIMINATE HARMFUL CHEMICALS SUCH AS ALCOHOL AND TOBACCO FROM MY DIET SO THAT I (AND THOSE AROUND ME) WILL BE HAPPIER AND HEALTHIER.**

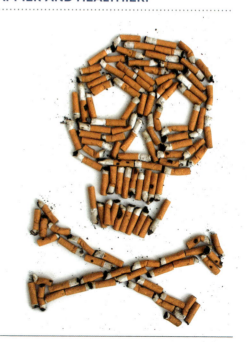

CHECK IT OUT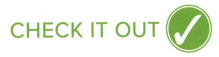

MY REASONS FOR NOT GOING VEGETARIAN HAVE INCLUDED:

- ☐ I LIKE EATING MEAT.
- ☐ VEGETARIANISM SEEMS UNNATURAL AND WEIRD.
- ☐ IT'S JUST A FAD THAT WILL PASS.
- ☐ MY FAMILY ALWAYS ATE MEAT, AND WE'RE FINE.
- ☐ GOING VEGETARIAN WOULD TAKE TOO MUCH OF MY TIME.
- ☐ I COULD NEVER GIVE UP _____ .
- ☐ WHAT I EAT IS NOBODY'S BUSINESS BUT MY OWN.
- ☐ I'M BASICALLY VEGETARIAN WITH JUST A FEW EXCEPTIONS.

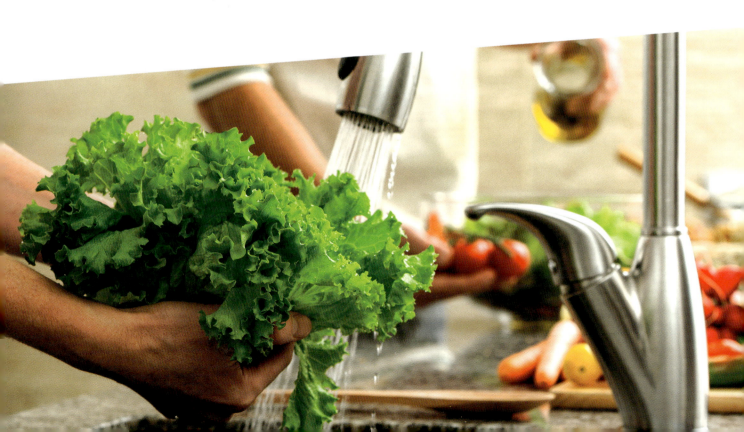

WHY BE VEGETARIAN?

Vegetarian can carry many meanings. For our purposes, vegetarian means eating and maintaining a plant-based diet without meat (that includes red meat, poultry and seafood). *Vegan* means abstaining from all animal products (this includes meat as well as eggs, milk and cheese).

"And the fear of you and the dread of you shall be on every beast of the earth, on every bird of the air, on all that move on the earth, and on all the fish of the sea." Genesis 9:2

Around eight billion animals are killed for food every year in the U.S. alone (about 900,000 per *hour).* Remember those beautiful pictures of grazing animals on green pastures so often seen in children's picture books? Animals used for food are usually raised in cramped confinement — a practice known as factory farming. Packed into cages with no free space, chickens have their beaks removed to keep them from pecking each other to death. The animals are pumped full of powerful drugs to kill diseases resulting from their filthy living conditions. These drugs (which people consume) also make the animals produce or grow faster than nature intended.

> *If slaughterhouses had glass walls, everyone would be vegetarian.*
>
> *Paul McCartney*

In *Old MacDonald's Factory Farm,* C. David Coates summarizes the killing game.

> Isn't man an amazing animal? He kills wildlife — birds, kangaroos, deer, all kinds of cats, coyotes, beavers, groundhogs, mice, foxes and dingoes — by the millions in order to protect his domestic animals and their feed. Then he kills his domestic animals by the billions and eats them. This in turn kills man by the millions, because eating all those animals leads to degenerative — and fatal — health conditions like heart disease, kidney disease and cancer. So then man tortures and kills millions more animals to look for cures for these diseases. Elsewhere, millions of other human beings are being killed by hunger and malnutrition because food they could eat is being used to fatten domestic animals. Meanwhile, some people are dying of sad laughter at the absurdity of man, who kills so easily and so violently and once a year sends out cards praying for Peace on Earth.

U.S. livestock produce 250,000 pounds of waste per second — 20 times as much as humans. A large feedlot produces as much waste as a big city, but without a sewage system. Animal waste washed into rivers and lakes increases nitrates, phosphates, ammonia and bacteria. The meat industry accounts for three times as much harmful organic waste as the rest of U.S. industries combined. According to ecological experts, becoming a vegetarian is the best thing one can do to heal the environment.

ADDITIONAL THOUGHTS ON VEGETARIANISM

1. HUNGER

- Number of people worldwide who will die as a result of undernutrition this year[6]: 8 million

- Number of children under 5 worldwide who will die as a result of undernutrition this year: 2.6 million

- Number of people who could be adequately fed using land freed for farming if Americans reduced their intake of meat by just 10%: 100 million

- Percentage of U.S. farmland devoted to beef productions: 56

2. CANCER

- Increased risk of breast cancer for women who eat meat daily compared to less than once a week: 3.8 times

- For women who eat eggs daily compared to once a week: 2.8 times

- Increased risk of fatal prostate cancer for men who consume meat, cheese, eggs and milk daily versus sparingly or not at all: 3.6 times

3. CHOLESTEROL

- Percentage of average U.S. man's risk of death from heart attack: 50

- Percentage risk of average U.S. man who eats no meat, dairy or eggs: 4

4. NATURAL RESOURCES

- Amount of water used for livestock production of all water used for all purposes in the U.S.: more than half

- Years the world's known oil reserves would last if every human ate a meat-centered diet: 13

- Years the reserves would last if human beings no longer ate meat: 260

5. ANTIBIOTICS

- Percentage of U.S. antibiotics fed to livestock: 55

- Percentage of staphylococci infections resistant to penicillin in 1960: 13

- Percentage resistant in 1988: 91

6. PESTICIDES

- Slaughtered animals in the U.S. tested for toxic chemical residues: fewer than 1 in 250,000

- Contamination of breast milk due to chlorinated hydrocarbon pesticides in animal products, found in meat-eating mothers versus non-meat eating mothers: 35 times higher

VEGETARIAN QUOTES

"The beef industry has contributed to more American deaths than all the wars of this century, all natural disasters, and all automobile accidents combined. If beef is your idea of 'real food for real people,' you'd better live real close to a real good hospital."

Neal D. Barnard, M.D.,
President, Physicians Committee
for Responsible Medicine

"Nothing will benefit human health and increase chances for survival of life on Earth as much as the evolution to a vegetarian diet."

Albert Einstein

To look closer into a nutritional vegetarian approach, refer to the resources at the end of this lesson.[6]

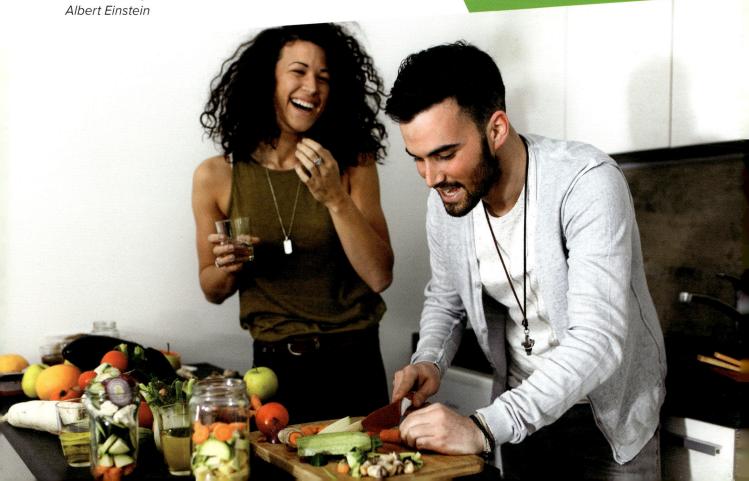

THE FULL PLATE DIET

What helps us most in turning the nutritional corner are practical, healthy tips and information. The following is from the excellent book *The Full Plate Diet*, by Stuart A. Seale, M.D., Teresa Sherard, M.D. and Diana Fleming, Ph.D., LDN. (available on Amazon. com). The Full Plate Diet is based on the concept of adding more fiber foods to our plates to lose weight and stay healthy.

Consider:

- In the 1800s, the average American consumed only 10 pounds of sugar per year. Today it's 158 pounds. There is no fiber in sugar.

- The number of U.S. children who took pills for type 2 diabetes more than doubled from 2002 to 2005. Type 2 diabetes is linked to obesity.

- Obesity can shorten your life by 10 years. Obesity will soon surpass tobacco in the U.S. as the leading cause of cancer.

Joe has been on the Full Plate Diet for three years, increasing the amount of natural, fiber-rich foods in his diet. In his first year, he lost 90 pounds and has easily kept the weight off.

His favorite part of the Full Plate Diet is he never felt he was going hungry. "You aren't starving yourself, and you don't have to do 100 sit-ups per day. You're just learning a new way of thinking about food."

THE EXCHANGE

MORE THIS	LESS THAT
Oranges	Orange Juice
Brown Rice	White Rice
High-Fiber Tortillas	White Flour Tortillas
Whole-Grain Bread	White Bread
Almonds	Candy
Apples/Bananas	Cookies
Sweet Potatoes	White Potatoes
Berries	Brownies
Oatmeal	Eggs
Fruit Smoothies	Milk Shakes
Beans or Hummus Dips	Sour Cream Dip
Bran Muffins	Donuts
Fruit Sorbets	Ice Creams
Applesauce	Pudding
Beans and Salsa on Baked Potatoes	Butter and Sour Cream on Baked Potatoes

FULL PLATE TIPS FOR EATING OUT

A. **Don't starve yourself before going out to eat.** If you haven't eaten all day, you're much more likely to overeat.

B. **Divide your servings** in half and share with a friend, or ask the waiter to bring a to-go box when your food is served, so you can halve your portion before you start eating.

C. **Be creative.** An item anywhere on the menu can be used to create a new option. Many times in side dishes there will be high-fiber foods you can use to power-up your entree (for example, add steamed broccoli to your pizza or beans to your salad).

D. **Ask that your vegetables** be steamed, baked, roasted or grilled, not fried.

E. **Going out to eat does not require you to have dessert.** If you feel the need for something sweet, order fresh fruit.

TOP 55 FULL PLATE FIBER FOODS

Top Fruits: apples, bananas, blackberries, blueberries, guava, kiwis, mangoes, oranges, papaya, peaches, pears, raspberries, strawberries

Top Vegetables: avocados, beets, broccoli, carrots, corn, green cabbage, kale, romaine lettuce, spinach, sweet potatoes, tomatoes, zucchini

Top Beans and Peas: black beans, black-eyed peas, garbanzo beans, green beans, green peas, kidney beans, lentils, lima beans, navy beans, peas, pinto beans

Top Grains: brown rice, buckwheat groats, millet, oats, pearl barley, quinoa, rye flakes, wheat, whole-grain cornmeal, wild rice

Top Nuts and Seeds: almonds, brazil nuts, chia seeds, flaxseeds, hazelnuts (filberts), peanuts, pecans, pumpkin seeds, sunflower seeds, walnuts

Let food be your medicine and medicine be your food.

Hippocrates

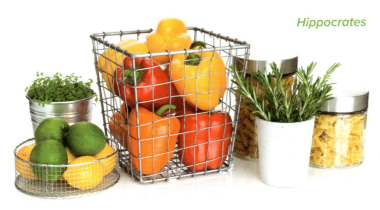

CHECK IT OUT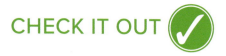

Rank the following from 1-8, with 1 being highest

WHAT DO YOU WANT MOST?

____ **MORE ENERGY**

____ **A LONG, HEALTHY LIFE**

____ **MY HEALTH PROBLEMS TO DISAPPEAR**

____ **TO LOSE WEIGHT WITHOUT BEING STRESSED ABOUT DIETING**

____ **MY FAMILY TO ESTABLISH GOOD EATING HABITS FOR THEIR LIVES**

____ **TO ENJOY LIFE DEEPLY AND LOVINGLY**

____ **NIGHTS FULL OF RESTFUL, REJUVENATING SLEEP**

____ **BETTER, CLEARER THINKING**

This is a difficult exercise, isn't it? Circle your top choice. (Apply it to your nutrition goal at the end).

BALANCED BEST

To maintain a balanced nutritional approach we can choose God's guidelines. However, situations may arise where it's difficult to follow those guidelines because of factors outside our control. In these moments we can feel confident about simply doing our "balanced best" and asking God for His blessing.

For example, if you are not willing to cut out meat entirely, but may be open to reducing your meat intake, try this approach:

- Start by replacing one meat item with a vegetable alternative each day

- Reduce the number of days a week you eat meat

- Consider buying organic, grass-fed, local meats that are raised humanely without antibiotics

We don't need to make a big scene about our diet. Be grateful and be humble. Twice, Jesus told His disciples to eat what was set before them.

"Whatever house you enter, first say, 'Peace to this house.' And if anyone is there who shares in peace, your peace will rest on that person; but if not, it will return to you. Remain in the same house, eating and drinking whatever they provide, for the laborer deserves to be paid. Do not move about from house to house. Whenever you enter a town and its people welcome you, eat what is set before you." Luke 10:5-8

We do not experience the benefits of following God's best plan of nutrition when we are overly "consumed" with details. Let's shift the focus from *what* we eat to eating so that we can love better.

Where do you tend to see yourself on the nutrition-caring scale?

Apathetic   Balanced   Obsessed

HOW DO I GO ABOUT MAKING CHANGES?

The best way to make changes in your lifestyle is to take it in stages and focus on the positive. Start by adding more fiber, fruits and vegetables rather than simply taking away all of the things you shouldn't be eating. Bad habits are usually squeezed out, not tweezed out. As you increase the positives, the negatives will seem to go away on their own.

Small changes can add up to big results. Along the way, you are likely to have set-backs, as with anything in life. No matter what your challenge, you can have a fresh start. Having support and a plan will make a positive impact on your journey. Pray to God for strength to achieve your goal, reach out to someone you trust that will keep you accountable or visit a licensed professional for counseling and support.

A mill worker was 100 pounds overweight and wanted to lose weight, but was too embarrassed to attend the nutrition classes his employer was offering. So the man went to see the class presenter in her office.

"Would you help me lose weight?" he asked.

"Of course," she said. "First, write down everything you eat each day of the week.

He brought the list back to her the next week. She looked it over and then asked him to eat one fruit every day in the coming week.

He said to her, "What about the half-pound of fudge I eat every day?"

She said, "Don't worry about that. It will take care of itself."

And it did. In the coming weeks the man noticed he craved more and more fruits and vegetables and had a decreasing desire for those foods he was in the habit of eating. The man went on to eating fruit at virtually every meal, and achieved success in his goal of losing weight.

Balance is key. Focus on taking one positive step at a time.

"For the earth yields crops by itself: first the blade, then the head, after that the full grain in the head."
Mark 4:28

LIVING BREAD AND WATER

"And Jesus said to them, 'I am the bread of life. He who comes to Me shall never hunger, and he who believes in Me shall never thirst.'" John 6:35

When we think about the ultimate nutrition, we arrive (as always with ultimate issues) at Jesus of Nazareth. Jesus forever satisfies our needs.

We don't need another super chef as much as we need a Savior, a person who can rescue us from meaninglessness and raise our dry bones from the sweating earth. Only One can do that.

"Jesus answered and said to her, 'If you knew the gift of God, and who it is who says to you, give Me a drink, you would have asked Him, and He would have given you living water.'" John 4:10

Sometimes it's astonishing how little we think of Jesus. If it was your earthly father who had been betrayed by a traitor, beaten senseless, tried and found innocent, then spiked to a tree and left to die, and if he did it all to take your place so that *you could live,* do you think you would be saying glibly, "Yes, I've heard about my father"? Would you not brim with tears each time you thought of him? Could you shrug it off if someone spoke poorly of him, or would you speak up indignantly in his defense? Would you forget about him — ever?

Jesus, however, thinks so much of us He has been "fasting" for close to 2,000 years.

"But I say to you, I will not drink of this fruit of the vine from now on until that day when I drink it new with you in My Father's kingdom." Matthew 26:29

This is a small preview of the welcome banquet that awaits every believer in Christ. What a celebration that will be!

"He brought me to the banqueting house, and His banner over me was love." Song of Solomon 2:4

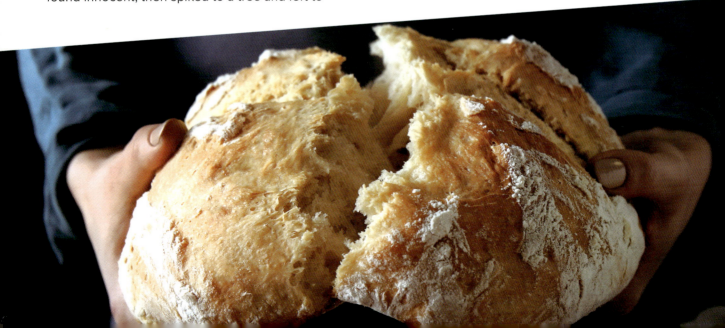

WILL WE EVER EAT OF THE TREE OF LIFE?

"He who has an ear, let him hear what the Spirit says to the churches. To him who overcomes I will give to eat from the tree of life, which is in the midst of the Paradise of God." Revelation 2:7

"Who is it that overcomes the world but he who believes that Jesus is the Son of God?" 1 John 5:5

God gave us perfection in the Garden of Eden. He graciously provided each gift of CREATION: Choice, Rest, Environment, Activity, Trust in God, Interpersonal Relationships, Outlook and Nutrition. Once again, God will recreate the paradise of Eden for all His believers on the new earth.

God wants you to choose His side and to abide with Him forever. When it all comes around, and this great controversy between good and evil is finished, like Adam and Eve we will taste the fruit from the Tree of Life. We will live forever with our Creator.

Do you long to experience freedom, joy and peace in an unending friendship with God? Do you wish to bring healing and hope to our hurting world? Do you want to live in the new earth with no more hatred, fear or suffering?

"And God will wipe away every tear from their eyes; there shall be no more death, nor sorrow, nor crying. There shall be no more pain, for the former things have passed away." Revelation 21:4

"For by grace you have been saved through faith, and that not of yourselves; it is the gift of God." Ephesians 2:8

We invite you to accept Jesus as your Savior, to live with His Spirit and to love your whole life. You are also humbly invited to connect with a community of believers at your local church.

"Behold, now is the acceptable time; behold, now is the day of salvation." 2 Corinthians 6:2

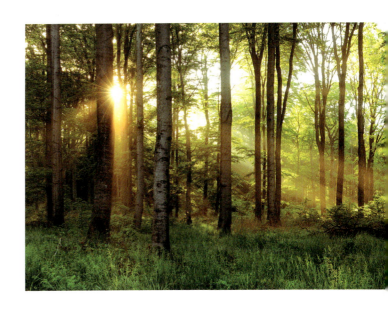

CREATION LIFE

NUTRITION

LIFE APPLICATION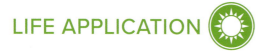

Take a moment to reflect on this CREATION Life study on nutrition.

WHAT PRINCIPLES HAVE YOU LEARNED THAT YOU WANT TO APPLY IN YOUR LIFE?

....

....

....

....

....

....

NOW, CREATE A PERSONAL GOAL FOR YOUR HEALTH AND NUTRITION.

....

....

....

....

....

....

....

Examples of goals for nutrition:

My goal is to eat at least one more fruit or vegetable a day than I am eating now. I will do this for a week. Then the next week I'll add one more, until I am eating five fruits and vegetables a day.

My goal is to drink eight glasses of purified water a day.

My goal is to eat something for breakfast each day this week. Next week, I'll eat two healthy items each day for breakfast, and continue this until it's my habit to eat a healthy, well-balanced breakfast.

My goal is to stop drinking alcohol, starting now.

My goal is to begin a vegetarian diet. I'll follow the Full-Plate Diet for at least one month. This means eating at least 25 grams of fiber each day.

"The Lord bless you and keep you; the Lord make His face shine upon you, and be gracious to you; the Lord lift up His countenance upon you, and give you peace."
Numbers 6:24-26

Eat less. Exercise more.

World's shortest diet book

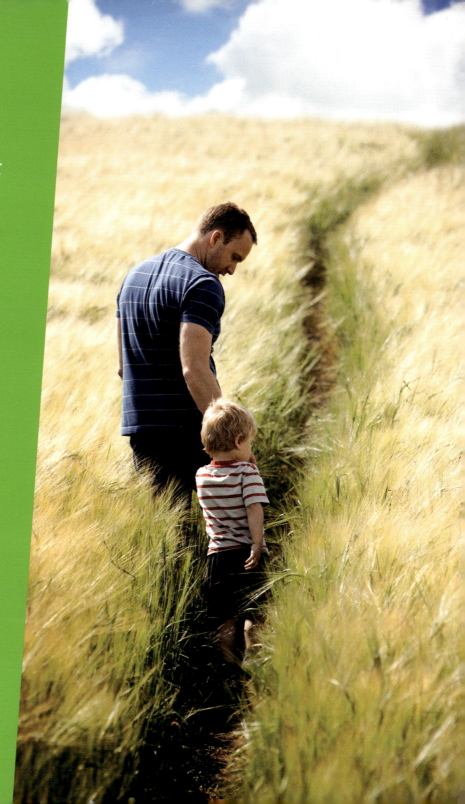

My Prayer: Yes, Jesus, please help me to walk every step of the way with You.

SMALL GROUP DISCUSSION QUESTIONS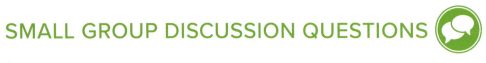

1. WHAT NUTRITIONAL HABIT WOULD MOST LIKELY SET YOU FREE?

    ....

    ....

2. READ DANIEL 1:1-20. HOW DOES THIS ANCIENT "DANIEL DIET" RELATE TO US TODAY?

    ....

    ....

3. DID YOU FEEL THIS SESSION WENT OVERBOARD IN "BASHING" ANYTHING?
    (ALCOHOL, TOBACCO, MEAT, CHEETOS?) EXPLAIN WHY YOU FEEL THIS WAY.

    ....

    ....

4. WHICH INFORMATION IN THE SESSION MADE THE GREATEST IMPACT ON YOU?

    ....

    ....

5. SHARE ONE OF YOUR NUTRITION GOALS. WHAT WILL HELP YOU
    EXPERIENCE SUCCESS IN REACHING THIS GOAL?

    ....

    ....

6. WHICH OF THE EIGHT PARTS OF CREATION LIFE WAS YOUR FAVORITE? WHY DID IT RANK SO HIGH?

....

....

....

....

7. THIS IS OUR FINAL SESSION. HOW WOULD YOU DESCRIBE THE CREATION LIFE EXPERIENCE? WHAT CAN WE DO TO CONTINUE OUR EXPERIENCE TOGETHER?

....

....

....

....

....

....

....

....

....

....

NOTES

CHOICE

1. Benton, P. (1984). *Grandma Wears Running Shoes*. Concerned Communications: Arroyo Grande, California.

2. As you pursue your choice to make your marriage (or dating relationship) better, we recommend *The Five Love Languages* by Gary Chapman.

3. Langer, E. J., & Rodin, J. (1976, August). Effects of choice and enhanced personal responsibility for the aged: A field experiment in an institutional setting. *Journal of Personality and Social Psychology, 34*(2), 191-198.

ENVIRONMENT

1. Ainsleigh, H. G. (1993, January). Beneficial effects of sun exposure on cancer mortality. *Prevention Medicine*, 22(1), 132-140.

ACTIVITY

1. Carson, B. with Murphey, C. (1992). *Think Big*. Hagerstown, MD: Review and Herald Publishing Association.

2. Maguire E., Frith C., Burgess N., et al. Knowing where things are: Parahippocampal involvement in encoding objects locations in virtual large scale space. *Journal of Cognitive Neuroscience,* 1998 Jan;10(1): 61-76.

3. Matthews, R. (1996) Importance of breakfast to cognitive performance and health. *Perspectives in Applied Nutrition,* 3(3), 204-212.

TRUST IN GOD

1. Cooper, D. (1995). *Living God's Love*. Nampa, ID: Pacific Press Publishing.

INTERPERSONAL RELATIONSHIPS

1. Sosa, R., Kennel, J., et al. (1980). The effect of a supportive companion on perinatal problems, length of labor and mother-infant interactions. *New England Journal of Medicine,* 303, 597-600.

2. Resnick, M., et al. (1997). Protecting adolescents from harm: Findings from the national longitudinal study on adolescent health. *Journal of the American Medical Association,* 278(10), 823-832.

3. Luks, A., & Payne, P. (1991). *The Healing Power of Doing Good: The health and spiritual benefits of helping others*. New York: Fawcett Columbine.

OUTLOOK

1. Adler, R., & Towne, N. (2010). *Looking Out/Looking In*. Fort Worth: Harcourt Brace Jovanovich.

2. Myers, D.G. (1980, May). The inflated self. *Psychology Today,* 16.

3. Emmons, R. A., & McCullough, M. E. (2003). Counting blessings versus burdens: An experimental investigation of gratitude and subjective well-being in daily life. *Journal of Personality and Social Psychology*, 84(2), 377-389.

4. Singer, B. (1974). The future-focused role-image. In A. Toffler (Ed.), *Learning for Tomorrow: The role of the future in education*. New York: Vintage Books.

5. (Sample) Our Family Values

   Maintain loving friendship with God first.
   Be honest and trustworthy.
   Work at holding a patient, positive, teachable outlook.
   Deeply respect life and environment.
   Maximize and risk God-given talents.
   Live healthy lives.
   Pray with all our mind, heart, soul, and strength.
   Use time responsibly.
   Practice courtesy, generosity, and service toward all people.

NUTRITION

1. Anderson, J. W., Smith, B. M., & Gustafson, N. J. (1994). Health benefits and practical aspects of high-fiber diets. *The American Journal of Clinical Nutrition,* 59(5), 12425-12475.

2. Allam, A. H., Thompson, R. C., Wann, L. S., Mlymoto, M. I., & Thomas, G. S. (2009). Computed tomographic assessment of atherosclerosis in ancient Egyptian mummies. *JAMA,* 302 (19), 2091-2094.

3. Matthews, R. (1996). Importance of breakfast to cognitive performance and health. *Perspectives in Applied Nutrition,* 3(3), 204-212.

4. Sources: WHO/WPRO – Smoking Statistics 28 May 2002. World Health Organization. The Health Consequences of Smoking: A Report of the Surgeon General 2004. Dept. Of Health and Human Resources – Centers for Disease Control and Prevention. The Health. Consequences of Involuntary Exposure to Tobacco Smoke: A Report of the Surgeon Generals 04 Jan 2007. U.S. Dept. of Health and Human Services.

5. UNICEF (2011). Levels and trends in child mortality. The statistics following are gathered from numerous sources. Please conduct your own research on reasons to go vegetarian.

6. Resources to get started:

   - *Vegetarian Beginner's Guide* by the editors of Vegetarian Times
   - *Become a Vegetarian in Five Easy Steps* by Christine H. Beard
   - *Complete Idiot's Guide to Being Vegetarian* by Suzanne Havala and Robert Pritikin
   - *Fix-It-Fast Vegetarian Cookbook* by Heather Houck Reseck
   - *Seven Secrets Cookbook* by Neva and Jim Brackett
   - *Refresh: Contemporary Vegan Recipes from the Award-Winning Fresh Restaurants* by Ruth Tal with Jennifer Houston
   - *The Perfectly Contented Meat-Eater's Guide to Vegetarianism* (a beginning guide with a huge dose of humor) by Mark Warren Reinhardt